A POWERFUL, DRUG-FREE PLAN TO QUIET
YOUR FEARS AND OVERCOME YOUR ANXIETY

the chemistry of calm

Settle your mind • Reclaim healthy emotions
Stop worrying and start fully living!

HENRY EMMONS, M.D.

author of *The Chemistry of Joy*

"Henry Emmons is a skilled and gifted physician who blends the best of Western science with complementary medicine and Eastern approaches to well-being. He holds it all together in the heart of a healer, and offers us his insights and practical advice in clear, graceful, and compelling prose. The 'calm' this book will help you achieve is not about going to sleep: it's about waking up!"

—Parker J. Palmer, author of *A Hidden Wholeness,*
The Courage to Teach, and *Let Your Life Speak*

THE
CHEMISTRY
OF
CALM

A Powerful, Drug-Free Plan to Quiet
Your Fears and Overcome Your Anxiety

Henry Emmons, M.D.

A TOUCHSTONE BOOK
Published by Simon & Schuster

New York   London   Toronto   Sydney

Touchstone
A Division of Simon & Schuster, Inc.
1230 Avenue of the Americas
New York, NY 10020

This publication contains the opinions and ideas of its author. It is intended to provide helpful and
informative material on the subjects addressed in the publication. It is sold with the understanding that
the author and publisher are not engaged in rendering medical, health, or any other kind of personal
professional services in the book. The reader should consult his or her medical, health or other competent
professional before adopting any of the suggestions in this book or drawing inferences from it.

The author and publisher specifically disclaim all responsibility for any liability, loss or risk,
personal or otherwise, which is incurred as a consequence, directly or indirectly, of the use
and application of any of the contents of this book.

First Touchstone trade paperback edition October 2010

TOUCHSTONE and colophon are registered trademarks of Simon & Schuster, Inc.

For information about special discounts for bulk purchases,
please contact Simon & Schuster Special Sales at 1-866-506-1949
or business@simonandschuster.com.

The Simon & Schuster Speakers Bureau can bring authors to your live event.
For more information or to book an event contact
the Simon & Schuster Speakers Bureau at 1-866-248-3049
or visit our website at www.simonspeakers.com.

Designed by Ruth Lee-Mui

Manufactured in the United States of America

5   7   9   10   8   6

Library of Congress Cataloging-in-Publication Data
Emmons, Henry.
The chemistry of calm : a powerful, drug-free plan to quiet your fears
and overcome your anxiety / by Henry Emmons
p. cm.
"A Touchstone Book"
Includes bibliographical references and index.
1. Anxiety—Alternative treatment—Popular works. I. Title.
RC531.E45 2011
616.85'223—dc22

2010024797

ISBN 978-1-4391-2906-7
ISBN 978-1-4391-4953-9 (ebook)

Contents

Part One

Build a Strong Foundation

Part Two

Awaken to Equanimity

Part Three

Understand Your Body-Mind

PART ONE

Build a Strong Foundation

The Promise of Tranquility

Why Anxiety Hurts, and How You Can Fix It

"I'M HAVING round two of PTSD. I haven't slept in seven months!"

Meeting me for the first time, Catherine slumped in her chair with fatigue, yet her body was so tense and restless that she could not stop moving. What bothered her most was the ceaseless movement of her mind, so locked in activity that it allowed her no rest, not even in sleep. "I've tried everything I've been told to do, and nothing has worked. I'm afraid I'll never come out of this. Is there any hope for me?"

Catherine's life had been entirely halted by anxiety. Nine years earlier, she had experienced a similar episode that left her paralyzed by fear. Then, too, she couldn't sleep well for months. She found sleeping medications to be helpful at that time. But now, reeling from her diagnosis of cancer just seven months ago, nothing was helping. She had tried half a dozen medications, yet slept only three to four hours per night. She could not turn off the cascade of fear, and despite trips to a sleep center and several doctors, she had lost any hope of improvement.

"I know it seems like it will never end," I told her, "but this is only temporary." I explained to Catherine that she was actually a very resilient person who normally enjoyed good health. Her fear switch was just locked in the on position right now, and it was keeping her stress hormones so high that she couldn't sleep. "We need to find some things to calm that down, and to get you sleeping again," I reassured her. "If you can get some sleep, I'm confident that you'll feel a whole lot better within a few days. Then we can look at ways to keep this from happening again."

And it was true. This bout with anxiety started when she learned that she had cancer, but the cancer was successfully treated and her prognosis was good. It's entirely normal to feel scared when one gets such a diagnosis, but for some reason her body and mind were unable to shut down that automatic stress reaction as they should have. And since she couldn't sleep, there was very little chance that they would do so.

I told Catherine to take a combination of supplements that I thought would calm her nervous system and help her sleep. I believed this to be the key to turning things around for her. She began using B vitamins, magnesium, and 5-HTP twice daily, along with tryptophan and a melatonin complex at night. Sure enough, within five days she clearly began to feel better. "It's amazing, the calming feeling these supplements give me. And the antianxiety medications I used before did nothing!" she told me, smiling for the first time since I had met her. Her sleep improved quickly and, as I expected, this allowed her mind to calm and her body to relax. The fear switch became unstuck, her stress hormones could return to normal, and she was able to turn her attention to getting her life back on track.

As so often happens, Catherine's entire life had been derailed by anxiety—not just once but twice. After her cancer diagnosis she had quit her job, left a community and lifestyle that she loved, and moved back in with her parents, who could help care for her. Though she was grateful to have her parents' support, she found herself socially isolated, as do so many who live with strong anxiety. She also feared that this spiral of anxiety would happen to her again. What could she do to prevent the cycle from starting all over again?

She decided to enter the Resilience Training Program. I started this program because our usual ways of treating anxiety and mood problems are so often insufficient. People like Catherine are frustrated with medications, want to learn things they can do for themselves, and desperately want to know how to prevent their debilitating bouts of anxiety from coming back again and again. They are looking for relief and are not finding it in the usual places. Resilience Training is a proven eight-week program that incorporates the latest science on diet, exercise, and nutritional supplements along with the best emotional self-care available—what I call the "psychology of mindfulness." Resilience Training is a step-by-step training in mental calmness and emotional wisdom, designed to help patients recover from and prevent relapse of anxiety, depression, and similar stress related problems. It has been effective even when medications are not—and in fact, many of my patients find they don't need to use traditional prescription antianxiety medication at all. In *The Chemistry of Calm*, I outline my entire approach to stress and anxiety problems, working with body and mind, heart and soul. We humans are complex beings, integrated and whole. When dealing with something as far-reaching as stress and anxiety can be, we need solutions that are as integrated and whole as we are.

Fear, worry, stress, and compulsivity, the unpleasant and unproductive states known collectively as anxiety, are even more common than depression. And anxiety states are increasingly frequent, especially in recent times. Like depression, the effects of anxiety extend beyond the body and mind to the entire being, affecting not only one's sense of well-being but also health, longevity, work productivity, relationships—the entire human condition.

As I explained to Catherine, fear itself is a normal, necessary part of being human. Like pain, it is a useful, even indispensable signal that there is something in our environment that is threatening or simply needs our attention. The problem comes when something goes awry in an otherwise normal process—when the reaction becomes excessive or unyielding. Parts of the body-mind turn off, while other areas get locked in the on position, unable to shut down even after the threat, if there ever was one, is long past. Catherine, for example, had a real scare with her cancer diagnosis. But it was a curable form of cancer that left her at no greater risk than anyone else. The problem was that she could not turn off her fear response.

Genetics plays a role in determining who gets an anxiety disorder, what type it is (e.g., worry, compulsive anxiety, or avoidant anxiety), and its severity. Genetic variability evolves over many millennia, yet we know that the rates of anxiety disorders have skyrocketed in just the last century, not to mention the last decade. I believe this has to do partly with changes in lifestyle, diet, sleep and work patterns, and especially our relationship with stress. Our world is unquestionably complex and in some ways intimidating. Much of the problem, though, lies not with how things have changed outside of us but with our lack of a skillful means for dealing with a challenging world. Catherine, for example, could have spared herself a great deal of suffering if she'd had the ability to fully face the sense of vulnerability that washed over her during her first brush with anxiety nine years earlier. Instead, it lodged in her body, ready to pounce again when faced with another overwhelming stress.

The Chemistry of Calm outlines a clear, holistic program for coping with fear and anxiety in much the same way my first book, *The Chemistry of Joy*, offered steps for overcoming depression. This book focuses on ways to create innate health and resilience as a key to resolving anxiety in everyday life—from the ordinary to the extreme. My goal is to help you understand fear and anxiety through a holistic lens and learn practical, integrative solutions that draw from new science, effective self-care, and solid spiritual practices. As I hear from so many of my patients: "I don't want to rely on medication for the rest of my life. I just want to know what I can do for myself!" This book is meant to give you just that—effective things that you can do for yourself to reclaim the resilience that is your birthright.

The Age of Anxiety

In just a few decades, dramatic changes have occurred in our relationship to stress. There are many illnesses that are now associated with stress—and they have become epidemic in scope.

The issue is not that life is so much more stressful now than ever before—a brief look at history may convince us otherwise. Imagine, for example, how stressful it was in times past to routinely lose children to illness; to truly not know whether you and your family would survive the winter; to endure plague, the Civil War, or the Great Depression. But while life has always been stressful, there is something different about how it affects us today, or perhaps how we respond to it.

Likewise, anxiety and its various disorders are nothing new. The ancient Greeks, for example, described agoraphobia (literally "fear of the marketplace") even in their day, when some had such severe anxiety that they could not leave their homes. Yet the scientific evidence reinforces our perceptions that modern life is stressful in different ways than before, that anxiety disorders are on the rise, and that other chronic illnesses have become entwined with the stress response. The phrase "the age of anxiety" has been used before, but perhaps never more aptly than now.

Anxiety disorders are easily the most common mental illnesses, affecting nearly one in five adult Americans in any given year and 30 percent of people in the United States at some point in their lives.[1] That's more than forty million people per year who have a diagnosable anxiety condition—not to mention those whose suffering doesn't quite cross the threshold into illness. Anxiety disorders are estimated to cost the economy over $50 billion per year, mostly from lost productivity.[2] Other consequences include an increased rate of heart disease, suicide, or death by other physical causes.[3]

At the same time, we have witnessed in the Western world an explosion of other chronic diseases that apparently are affected by the stress response. Heart disease, Alzheimer's, chronic fatigue, high blood pressure, asthma, immune system diseases, and even cancer are linked to unhealthy levels of stress and the stress hormones. This problem is highlighted in a recent report by the Greater Boston Physicians for Social Responsibility *and* Science and Environmental Health Network. Titled "Environmental Threats to Healthy Aging," the report notes that while we live longer today than ever before, we are at increasing risk of developing neurodegenerative diseases. The report refers to the "Western disease cluster" (diabetes, obesity, hypertension, elevated blood lipids, and metabolic syndrome) as factors in the development and progression of various brain disorders.[4]

It's Not All in Your Head . . .

I don't see the mind, body, and spirit as separate things—they are just different reflections of a unified whole. But too often we focus on one and forget the others. The physical and emotional conditions of stress and anxiety have become the scourges of modern life, and they create a huge amount of suffering. What you do to relieve these in the mind also helps the body and spirit—and vice versa. Let's take a closer look at some of the different aspects of the stress/fear cycle, all of which we will address in the Resilience Training Program.

The Adrenal/Stress Response

The adrenal/stress response is the key to whether or not fear makes us sick. It is not that stress itself is bad. Studies show that short-term stress can even be good for us. But as the military has discovered, if the amount of stress is great enough, anyone can be broken down by it. Most of us, of course, don't experience severe stress in our day-to-day lives. But if your daily life is filled with constant, unremitting stress—if stress is ever present, like background noise—it can be destructive. Still, what determines how well you survive chronic stress is how you react to it and whether you are able to shut it down. Throughout this book you will learn how to protect your body from the corrosive effects of stress.

Brain on Fire: The Destructive Effects of Inflammation

Inflammation is supposed to be one of the ways by which the body protects itself. The redness and swelling that you see with an infection of the skin, for example, are signs that the immune system is doing its job, rallying the troops to the area to fight off the infection. Or if you injure your ankle, it too becomes red and swollen as extra blood and repair cells flow to the area to begin the process of healing.

But your own immune system can turn against you and become the very cause of the damage. Asthma is one example of this; rheumatoid arthritis is another. For reasons that may include genetics, environmental factors, or diet, the immune system is overreacting. Excessive inflammation of the airways causes them to swell and constrict, resulting in difficult breathing for the asthmatic. In rheumatoid arthritis, the joint itself is damaged because of the overdone inflammation response.

Yet there is an even more insidious side to inflammation. When it becomes systemic—that is, when it affects the whole body—then it causes strain on cells everywhere. And usually we don't even know it—it is silent. In recent years, systemic inflammation has been linked to a number of problems, including diabetes, cancer, Alzheimer's, Parkinson's, and heart disease.

I address inflammation in the Resilience Training Program because I think that if something is bad for the rest of the body, it is also bad for the brain. Systemic inflammation affects the whole body, after all, and it also puts a strain on brain cells. Indeed, many of my patients show signs of inflammation, and when they take measures to calm it, they also calm their anxiety and improve their mood. The reverse is also true—when they calm their mind through meditation and awareness practices, the stress response can shut down and so can their inflammation.

Starving in a World of Excess: Insulin Resistance and Metabolic Syndrome

Most of us in the developed world get an adequate (or excessive) amount of food each day. But from the point of view of the individual cells, there may be a serious lack of what is needed for the cells to do their all-important work. That lack can cause poor communication with other cells, low energy, lack of mental focus, and the inability to shut down the stress response.

There is a spectrum of problems caused by insulin resistance, from very mild trouble processing blood sugar (or blood glucose) to full-blown diabetes requiring the medication insulin. If the mild problems are not heeded and the condition progresses, it may evolve into metabolic syndrome, also known as pre-diabetes. This member of the "Western disease cluster" includes high blood pressure, elevated triglycerides, low HDL cholesterol, and inflammation.[5] It is often evidenced by an increase in belly fat. If the condition is not reversed, it can begin to cause lasting damage to the heart and nervous system. But for most people, it can be reversed.

The frequency of these problems has exploded in recent years, along with the rise in obesity. They are most likely caused by changes in diet—eating too much sugar or other highly refined carbohydrates—compounded by lack of physical activity. But what does this have to do with anxiety?

Anxiety, depression, and insomnia have all been associated with production of excess insulin.[6] The body produces more insulin when cells lose their ability to use the message that insulin gives them. This insulin resistance elevates inflammation and stress hormones.[7] In addition, excess insulin deprives the brain of its steady supply of glucose for fuel, so it sends off a strong alarm signal, further heightening the state of stress or anxiety.

. . . But Some of It Is in the Mind

We need to address problems occurring in the physical body because they so strongly impact the brain's ability to function well. But we still have to recognize the central importance of the thinking mind, especially in creating stress and anxiety. As Robert Sapolsky, a noted author and stress expert puts it, zebras don't get ulcers—they don't suffer from chronic stress.

But people do, and there are myriad problems associated with long-term stress. Why are we humans so susceptible to stress? Sapolsky says it is because "we've evolved to be smart enough to make ourselves sick."[8] Since our most obvious survival needs are taken care of, we have too much time on our hands—time to turn that intelligent mind against ourselves. In other words, we think, therefore we are stressed.

The Second Arrow

Buddhist psychology would agree with this. In the Buddhist view of the mind, we inadvertently harm ourselves through our own thinking. Buddhists use a battlefield image to describe this. A soldier may be injured in the course of battle, hit by an arrow. That is the risk of being a soldier. Likewise, we will inevitably experience pain or distress in the course of our lives. That is known as the "first arrow," and it is largely unavoidable. If we're in the game, so to speak, we run the risk of injury.

But imagine that same soldier taking a second arrow and shooting himself with it. Of course that wouldn't happen—yet that is just what we do when the thinking mind kicks into gear and we turn the seed of fear into something much larger through worry, regret, rumination, and the like. This is precisely what happened to Catherine. She began to think—and that's when her real trouble began.

We do not create such troublesome thoughts intentionally. No one really wants to suffer more. We aren't aware that we are doing this to ourselves and we don't know how to stop it. But we can become conscious and skilled at breaking out of this cycle, as hundreds of people have learned through the Resilience Training Program, and as you will learn to do, too.

Mind on Fire: The Destructive Potential of Mental Storms

We've all had them—times when our thinking takes off down dark alleys and we seem unable to stop it. We all know, from personal experience, that once the brain circuitry heats up, it becomes more intense and unpleasant—and increasingly hard to stop. And the storm tends to spread. Soon it is no longer confined to our thoughts. The emotions get involved, and then the rest of the body starts reacting and reinforcing the whole mess.

But while it may seem like we have little control over it, we can actually develop skills that help us to find a calm port in the storm. We can learn to steady the mind and work with the emotions so that they have less destructive force behind them. We can't completely avoid the storms, any more than we can avoid pain or stress. But there is a lot we can learn to do to soften their effects and to hold ourselves steady until the storm passes.

The Constricted Heart: The Tragic Result of Trauma and Fear

What do we do when we feel threatened or, worse yet, become traumatized? We protect ourselves automatically, doing whatever it takes. Very often that involves shutting ourselves down in some way, closing ourselves off from anything that might cause further fear or pain. That might not be such a bad strategy if we knew how to open up again when the threat was gone. But for various reasons, we don't. The emotional heart hardens, shrinks back, or becomes dulled—anything not to feel the pain or to be consumed by fear.

There is plenty to feel threatened by in this world. In the past few years, we have witnessed troubled children shooting other children in our schools, fanatical men flying jets into buildings, innocent lives torn apart by war not of their own making, vast economies crumbling under the weight of unchecked greed, soldiers coming home carrying the psychic wounds of war, and women and children the world over suffering the effects of abuse and neglect. What sane person would not feel anxious, stressed, or fearful? Why would you not want to close yourself off from this? What else can we do with these and the other, more personal tragedies that befall us every day?

It is interesting that the word *courage* comes from the Latin root *cor*, meaning "heart." To have courage is to take heart or, one might say, to reclaim the heart. This may sound vague or "soft," yet I find the mindfulness practices that I call "cultivating a good heart" to be among the most powerful, life-giving, and courageous acts I know. To live with some measure of acceptance, gratitude, forgiveness, and generosity, to find a level of openness and equanimity in the face of such fearful things—these are acts of great courage. And it is good medicine, too—we feel better when we live with a more open heart.

Isolation: We Are Not Meant for This

Simply put, we are not built for lives of separation. In my view, feeling disconnected is the number one reason for a loss of vitality, for living a sort of shadow life. And when I think of connection, I look at it in a very broad sense. Yes, it is important to have friends and ties to family and community. But there is also the connection with nature, which can be so life-giving. There is the relationship with ourselves, at all levels—caring enough about our body that we take care of it, accepting ourselves even with all of our past mistakes and present flaws, giving some time and attention to our inner lives. When we do that, we realize that we long for connection to something larger than ourselves—meaning, purpose, a relationship with the Divine.

Opening ourselves to these and other connections transforms

the dynamic of self-care. These are the things that not only keep us afloat—they make us bigger than ourselves. Meaningful connection enlarges our lives.

How to Use This Book

I wish it were otherwise, but millions and millions of people are in a state of depletion today. *The Chemistry of Calm* is intended as a guide to reclaiming your resilience, to moving from a state of stress, anxiety, or fear to a place of calm, balance, and equanimity. I will show you how to calm the fires of an overactive brain, endocrine system, or immune system. You will learn how to become skilled at working with your own thoughts and feelings so that they are once again allies, and not enemies, in your quest to live a more balanced and serene life. And you are also invited to go beyond good self-care, to begin a process of transformation and to claim for yourself the rich, vital, and courageous life that you long for.

The basis of *The Chemistry of Calm* is the Resilience Training Program. The program consists of seven steps, what I call the seven Roots of Resilience. In Part One, steps 1–3, we will focus on the physical body (including the brain) with lifestyle measures and integrative medical therapies. In Part Two, steps 4–7, we will turn to the inner aspects of resilience, to help you deal with difficult emotional states such as fear and anxiety.

The Roots of Resilience
1. **Balance your brain chemistry.** In chapters 4 and 5,
   you'll learn about proper diet, supplements, and even
   medications when needed.

2. **Manage your energy.** In chapter 6, you'll learn how exercise and moving your body can actually create more energy and better mental health.

3. **Align yourself with nature.** In chapter 7, you'll learn how to calm your sleep patterns and recharge your mind.

4. **Quiet your mind.** Chapter 8 describes the core practices of mindfulness: awareness of breathing and awareness of thought.

5. **Face your emotions.** In chapter 9 you will learn how to remain steady even if overcome by a "mental storm."

6. **Cultivate a good heart.** In chapter 10, you'll focus on opening your heart—cultivating self-acceptance, loving-kindness, generosity, and gratitude.

7. **Create deep connections.** In chapter 11, you'll contemplate the importance of connecting with others—developing a sense of belonging in the larger world.

Part Three gives more detailed background and the scientific underpinnings for the program. This final part of the book focuses on the clinical and scientific aspects of anxiety, including groundbreaking new research that gives hope and inspiration to all who suffer from stress and anxiety.

The suggestions in this book offer a promise that is both authentic and attainable. Over and over again we see people in our program leave behind a lifetime of struggle to find a degree of equanimity and fullness in their lives that they had not dreamed possible. Resilience is indeed within your reach.

Are You Ready?

We know from research on changing healthy behaviors that there is a wide spectrum of readiness—ranging from not yet ready at all to having already made the changes and simply needing to maintain them. And there is every gradation in between. Wherever you fall on that spectrum, I would encourage you to honestly accept that and be okay with it. There is no "right way" to do this program—or, for that matter, to live one's life. And I believe that there is something in this book for anyone who wants to live a life of greater freedom, fullness, and vitality.

If you are just thinking about it, you may want to start with Part Three to gather more background and understanding. Perhaps you will be informed and inspired enough to shift yourself a bit further toward taking action. If you are ready to make changes but not too sure about your level of commitment, you may want to read chapter 12 to help increase your sense of hope and derive more motivation from that. Then you can return to the program in Parts One and Two.

Some elements of building a foundation are relatively easy to do (such as sleeping more and taking supplements), and others require more committed focus (such as changing diet and exercising). I will provide a full spectrum of healthy options, from simple things you can begin today to profound practices that you can do for a lifetime. Start wherever you can, and build from there.

It is important to begin where you feel the most energy or have the greatest need. You can always go back to earlier sections later on—you will always want to have a firm physical foundation, after all. But whenever you are ready for a process of inner transformation, you may move on to Part Two. There you can learn to tame your mind and emotions and grow more and more fully into yourself.

2

A Brief History of Anxiety

Why We Are Stressed—and Why a Prescription May Not Be the Best Answer

JESSICA ADMITTED that she had always been "a little high-strung" and that worry was second nature to her. She was constantly on the lookout for what might be amiss, and sometimes she had trouble sleeping when her thinking mind became engaged. Still, for the first thirty years of her life, this was simply part of who she was, as likely to be helpful as it was annoying. She could even laugh along with her friends when they teased her about seeing what would go wrong before it happened. In fact, she was a great mother who anticipated her children's needs and potentially risky behaviors before they occurred. Responsible and attentive to detail, she was just the person you would want to do your legal work, which was how she had made a living before she became incapacitated by anxiety.

Her story began one year before she saw me, when anxiety turned suddenly from a trait into a serious problem. Like many Minnesotans, she dreaded the start of winter, or more specifically winter driving. Then one November day, as she drove her children to day care, it began to snow. As the snow fell, Jessica's tension rose.

In many ways, Jessica was perfectly suited for a circumstance like this. When great care was required, she was up to the task. So she was poised for danger—sitting upright, leaning forward, and tightly gripping the wheel. She was totally focused on the road ahead, scanning for anything amiss, keeping a safe distance from other cars and barely inching along. She was doing everything in her power to keep herself and her children safe.

As she cautiously entered an intersection, her car was suddenly slammed into from the side. She reacted quickly, becoming even more focused and alert than before. She stopped and secured the car, then immediately checked on her children. They were both crying in the backseat. She spoke soothingly to them as she did a quick scan to see if they were injured, but they appeared unhurt. She gathered them up in her arms, as if to protect them from further danger. Though she was not thinking about it, she was on high alert at that moment, in a state of stress but not really anxious. She acted instinctively and flawlessly. Her mind seemed clear and her decisions flowed effortlessly.

Before long, her attention turned to the car that had struck her. The other driver was an elderly man, and the growing crowd was attending to him. He had been unable to stop at the red light and had slid through the intersection into Jessica's car. The impact had left him dazed, and it appeared that he had hit his head. Jessica herself was very concerned about him, and it was a relief when the police and then an ambulance arrived.

They were all taken to the hospital as a precaution. Jessica was still hyperalert, her body stressed but her mind clear and focused. It wasn't until the doctors assured her that neither she nor her children were injured—and that the man from the other car had suffered only a mild concussion and he would likely be okay—that she began to relax.

Later that night, as she lay in bed replaying the events of the day, her real nightmare began. Her thinking mind kicked into gear. *What if my children had been really hurt? What if the elderly man has internal bleeding? What if he dies?* That fear really stuck in her mind, and she replayed it over and over. Before long, no amount of reassurance could convince her that he would be all right. From that seed of a thought sprang a whole year of growing fear—and a shrinking life.

Jessica's journey with fear is just beginning, and we'll return to it later. But already it illustrates some key lessons about fear and anxiety. One is that being anxious is not a sign of moral weakness or an issue of character. You could hardly find a more solid or more likeable person than Jessica. In fact, some of her life success could be attributed to her anxious nature. Anticipating what could go wrong made her a better parent and attorney. She could see every possible outcome, making it more likely that she would avoid pitfalls. And she could learn from things that did go awry. There can be value in rehearsing the future and reflecting on the past—at least up to a point.

Her car accident is an example of how fear has its benefits. The best thing she could have done while driving in the snow was to be vigilant, with all of her senses heightened. There was, in fact, danger, and she was right to be on guard for it. Stress, which has taken on a negative meaning in modern culture, is not altogether a bad thing. Her own reaction to stress helped her become more focused and action-oriented when she and her children needed it most.

The Evolution of Fear

It is clear that people are born with different temperaments, and that some of us, like Jessica, are born to worry. Anxious traits, along with illnesses such as panic disorder and obsessive-compulsive disorder (OCD), tend to run in families. They are in part genetic. This raises some obvious questions: Why would we have anxiety in our gene pool? Has evolution somehow favored genes for worry, panic, or compulsiveness? Why is fear woven so tightly into our biology?

There is a scientific discipline known as evolutionary psychology that studies these very questions and has concluded that fear is helpful for our survival. Like other core emotions, fear provided an adaptive advantage as we evolved. At its root, fear is the signal that tells us we are in danger and motivates our action to deal with it. Fear helps us anticipate and avoid danger. And when we can't avoid it, fear and the stress response that it triggers help us escape. If escape is not possible, then the stress response enables us to fight for our survival. As we saw with Jessica, it sharpens all of our senses and gives a laser-like focus to the mind. In that moment, everything else fades in significance, and we are totally intent upon safety—not only for ourselves but for others as well.[1]

Evolutionary psychology suggests that those with the most effective fear and avoidance mechanisms were the most likely to survive in the harsh environments of our ancestors. As humans banded together, the entire group's chances of survival were improved by having someone like Jessica in their tribe. It helped to have someone scanning the horizon, on the lookout for enemies or predators—someone whose level of vigilance was set a bit higher than most. And if this person's panic button went off quickly when danger was near, then he or she could alert others. A worrier is always thinking ahead—planning, for example, how to survive the winter. That could help ensure that everyone in the tribe secured adequate shelter. Or someone who was compulsive about gathering extra food and setting it aside for leaner times might benefit the whole family by doing so. When it comes to survival, there is a lot to be said for having a healthy dose of worry and fear.[2]

The Battle Against Fear

The study of evolution gives us a certain perspective on fear and anxiety, one that I believe helps us see it as an adaptive trait. But while evolution seems to have favored the development of anxious traits, human history has largely been unkind to those who have them. That has been especially true in the history of war, where fear itself is often considered the enemy.

Soldiers who could not successfully control their fear have been treated harshly throughout military history. The ancient Greeks believed that a soldier's moral character was reflected by how well he controlled his fear in battle. Those who kept a tight lid on it were considered heroes, while those who did not were called cowards. The Greeks believed so strongly in this that they chose not to modernize their battle techniques for hundreds of years, believing that to do so might blur the distinction between bravery and cowardice. Such beliefs have persisted into modern times. During the American Civil War, vast numbers of soldiers became incapacitated by anxiety. Many of them were publicly shamed for being "cowardly" by being branded or tattooed.[3]

World War I became known for its trench warfare and soldiers' prolonged exposure to shelling. This produced huge numbers of soldiers unable to fight for psychological reasons—up to 40 percent of battlefield casualties by some estimates.[4] But at the time, doctors thought that the concussive effects of the constant shelling somehow damaged the nervous system—hence the name *shell shock*. It was not yet understood to be an emotional reaction.[5] Many of these impaired soldiers, labeled as weak and inferior, were initially court-martialed or dishonorably discharged.

But soldiers were a valuable resource, and as the numbers of psychiatric casualties grew, there was increasing pressure to treat them and get them back on the battlefield. For the most part, the treatments available at the time were not very effective. There was only one factor that correlated strongly with their ability to return to battle—the degree to which they felt a close emotional bond to their fellow soldiers.[6]

By the start of World War II, medical experts tried to remove the stigma from what was previously known as "combat neurosis." They called it simply "exhaustion" and began treating the soldiers with rest. They had learned the lessons from the previous war and set up hospitals close to the front so that they would remain near their comrades.

Stigmas don't go away easily. In a well-known incident in 1943, General George S. Patton visited a hospital and came upon a soldier who had been diagnosed with "psycho-neurosis anxiety." This turned out to be the wrong diagnosis—he was later discovered to have dysentery. Patton asked him what was wrong and the soldier, filled with shame, replied, "I guess I just can't take it." Patton was infuriated. He yelled and slapped the soldier, then physically threw him out of the tent. He later issued a memo saying, "Such men are cowards" and should be court-martialed.[7] Luckily, that order wasn't followed, because there were over half a million American soldiers unable to fight during World War II because of "psychiatric collapse"—more than the number killed in action or disabled by any other cause.[8]

Such high numbers of stress-related casualties challenged the view that breakdown in battle occurred because one was weak or lacking in courage. Not only were the numbers staggering, but also many of the disabled had been known for acts of heroism both before and after being overcome by fear. It was beginning to dawn on military and medical leaders that this sort of anxiety reaction is simply what happens to normal people who are exposed to too great a strain. In a 1946 article, the authors concluded, "There is no such thing as 'getting used to combat.' . . . men will break down in direct relation to the intensity and duration of their exposure. Thus psychiatric casualties are as inevitable as gunshot and shrapnel wounds in warfare."[9]

With the Vietnam War came a new term to describe this phenomenon—post-traumatic stress disorder. This was also the war where PTSD was no longer hidden from the public. The entire nation witnessed the return of soldiers experiencing flashbacks, addicted to drugs, or otherwise suffering from the psychological wounds they carried. Prominent television coverage and popular movies helped weave these images into the American psyche. In an article published in *Science* in 2006, researchers from Columbia University reviewed military records and concluded that 18.7 percent of Vietnam vets suffered from PTSD. What's more, about half of those still had symptoms nearly fifteen years after the war had ended.[10] It was becoming clear that the effects of extreme stress not only impacted one in the short term, but also could cause long-lasting, sometimes disabling symptoms. And the effects of trauma extend well beyond psychological suffering. A study of U.S. army veterans thirty years after their military service ended showed that those with PTSD die at twice the rate of veterans the same age without PTSD.[11]

At this moment in history, soldiers are facing the same age-old problems from the stress of warfare and are still not getting sufficient help. Recent surveys suggest that 25–30 percent of soldiers returning from Iraq and Afghanistan suffer from a mental disorder, and that for most of them this is the direct effect of stress. Yet because of stigma, less than half of them seek help—and those who do seek help often find that the resources for treatment simply aren't available.[12]

The Phenomenon of Hysteria

The history of combat-related anxiety has been largely confined to men, at least until recently. And for centuries the notion of "hysteria" was thought to apply only to women. This idea first took hold in ancient Greece. Hippocrates, the "father of medicine" whose healing oath is revered to this day, used the term *hysteria* to describe overwhelming fear, sometimes accompanied by unexplained physical symptoms or loss of self-control. He believed that hysteria was caused by the uterus (*hystera* in Greek) moving upward and compressing the diaphragm, lungs, and heart. The ancient Greeks believed that this occurred because of sexual inactivity or frustration. Surprisingly, these ideas persisted through the eighteenth century, when the famous French psychiatrist Philippe Pinel and others suggested marriage and childbearing as a treatment for hysteria.[13]

In the late 1800s hysteria became a phenomenon in Europe. It was still associated exclusively with women, and many of them were put onstage to demonstrate their symptoms in large clinical gatherings. The public largely saw these women as malingerers and viewed the hypnotists and others who treated them as frauds. But then a French physician, Jean-Martin Charcot, began to treat hysteria as an organic disease worthy of scientific study. He believed it to be genetic, recognized that both physical and emotional factors were at play, and saw that it could occur in men as well as women. He also realized that traumatic experiences could trigger the illness.[14] Charcot was considered to be one of the preeminent physicians of his time, and he lent an aura of credibility to the condition. But his own fame and stature could not protect him from a public backlash. It became widely rumored that the demonstrations that had so fascinated Parisians involved nothing more than suggestible women who were following a script—playacting, with no real illness. Charcot's work, the first to begin to see anxiety reactions in their full scope, became tainted. By the end of his life, he regretted ever having gotten into this line of research.[15]

Among those who traveled to study with Charcot were the great American psychologist William James and an Austrian neurologist named Sigmund Freud. Freud, who suffered from anxiety himself, concluded that hysteria had its roots in psychological trauma during childhood. His theories took hold in American psychiatry, and the term *hysteria* came to mean "emotionally charged situations . . . symbolic of underlying conflicts." But unlike his colleagues who believed it to be a sign of psychological weakness, Freud said that hysteria occurred in "people of the clearest intellect, strongest will, greatest character, and highest critical power."[16]

William James was even more empathic when he wrote: "Amongst the many victims of medical ignorance clad in authority the poor hysteric has hitherto fared the worst; and her gradual rehabilitation and rescue will count among the philanthropic conquests of our generation."[17]

Yet here we are, over a century later, still working under a cloud of ignorance and stigma regarding the condition broadly known as anxiety. Perhaps understanding the relationship between anxiety and stress may help us out of this dilemma.

The Rise of Stress, the Fall of Resilience

Prior to 1914 the word *stress* was an engineering term, as in the force placed on a structure that causes it to break down in some way. Then

Walter Cannon used *stress* in a biomedical sense when he described the "fight-or-flight syndrome" and the stress response.[18] A physiologist, he viewed the fight-or-flight reaction as the body's emergency response, shifting blood flow so that energy could go where it was really needed (like the heart and skeletal muscles) and conserve it where it wasn't needed (such as the gut or the extremities). If you're in a life-or-death situation, you don't need to digest food or keep your hands warm—you need to have your wits about you and be able to use your muscles to get out of there fast, or fight your way out if you have to. Cannon later described how epinephrine (also known as adrenaline), norepinephrine, and the sympathetic nervous system worked together to create the stress response. Interestingly, Cannon viewed stress positively, and in *The Wisdom of the Body* he wrote about humans' innate ability to handle all kinds of stresses. In his view, the stress response is a normal and essential reaction to threats, like what Jessica experienced while driving in the snow, and which everyone displays from time to time.

Just a few years after Cannon defined the fight-or-flight syndrome, an endocrinologist named Hans Selye realized that stress wasn't *always* normal. Under some conditions, stress could make a person sick. Selye was working with rats in the laboratory and realized that when the rats were exposed to chronic stress they developed ulcers and their immune tissues shrank, while their adrenal glands got bigger.

Further study suggested that the body responds similarly to all sorts of stress, and Selye described three stages of the stress response. First, there is an alarm stage, like what Cannon called the fight-or-flight syndrome. Next is what he called adaptation, or "resistance," when the body rises to the challenge and adapts to the stressful conditions. For example, we become more resistant to disease as the immune system kicks into high gear. During this phase, it is easy to feel complacent or invulnerable, to think, "I can handle it," because we feel good. But that doesn't last.

If the stress goes on long enough, then the third stage—which Selye called "exhaustion"—will inevitably set in. And then we are more susceptible to illness. Selye saw this third stage as a state of depletion, where the stress hormones that have been so dutifully produced for so long begin to run out. As it turns out, though, the problems with chronic stress occur not because of depletion, as Selye thought, but because the stress response itself becomes damaging.[19]

We are resilient beings by nature. Everyone has a different degree of stress tolerance, and indeed, some can "handle it" for what seems like a long time. It is great to be so resilient, but too often it allows the stressful situation to go on and on. Ironically, that very resilience gives us the option of not doing anything about the stress. If allowed to go unchecked, it will create physical problems beyond the unpleasant emotions of fear and anxiety. The cycle of stress tends to perpetuate itself, to get locked in place as the mind and body keep spinning a web of self-injury.

The stakes are too high to allow this to go on unchecked. We have to learn to recognize the patterns of stress and anxiety and intervene intelligently. To me, that means seeing our complexity and wholeness and finding solutions that are as whole and complex as we are. Yet it is human nature to look for an easier way to relieve our suffering. For much of human history, that effort has been through chemicals.

The Search for a Cure

As long as intoxicating substances have been available, people have turned to them to alleviate fear and anxiety. Alcohol has been around for at least ten thousand years, and to this day it is the choice of millions to calm their own anxiety. Opium, the "joy plant," goes back as far as 3400 BC in Mesopotamia in its use as a sedative. And as early as

2000 BC, tribes living on the Russian steppes used psychoactive mushrooms to reduce their fears.[20]

Then, in 1805, the modern era of psychopharmacology was born. Morphine (named after Morpheus, the Greek god of dreams) was isolated from opium and was lauded as a great advance, considered far more reliable and safer than opium. This is a common theme repeated with nearly every discovery of the next great medicine for anxiety: there is an initial excitement, it is lauded as being more safe and effective than its predecessor, it becomes widely used, and then it is realized that there are in fact many problems with it, often involving addiction and withdrawal. Morphine itself was used not only for pain relief but also as a "cure" for opium and alcohol addiction, only to be found later to be highly addictive itself.

Since then, there has been a succession of similar hopeful cures. Chloral hydrate, manufactured in 1832, became the Prozac of its day—the rock star of psychotropic drugs. Used to treat anxiety and insomnia, it was still prescribed as a sleep remedy for more than 150 years after it was discovered. Bromine became the next big thing in 1857, followed by barbital, the first of the barbiturates. It was so successful a drug that there were dozens of other barbiturates developed in the early 1900s, many of which became household names, like *phenobarbital*.[21]

In the middle of the twentieth century psychopharmacology became truly big business, in large part due to the great desire to reduce anxiety. In the 1960s, the benzodiazepines were developed, and were welcomed as a more effective and safer treatment than opium and the barbiturates. Librium, Dalmane, Xanax, Ativan, Klonopin, and others were released as each drug company tried to match the phenomenal success of Valium, the most-prescribed drug in America by the late 1960s—a position it held for more than a decade. In the 1970s, it was estimated that nearly a quarter of American men and over one-third of women were taking a psychoactive drug, most often a benzodiaz-epine.[22] That has changed since the mid-1980s, for two reasons: it became clear that they were in fact highly addictive (and often lost their effectiveness) with long-term use, and Prozac was introduced in the United States in 1988.

In our lifetimes, there has not been anything quite like the phe-nomenon of Prozac. Books and songs have been written about it. Mil-lions upon millions of people have taken Prozac, a selective serotonin reuptake inhibitor (SSRI), along with its cousins Zoloft, Celexa, Paxil, Luvox, and Lexapro. They are used for a host of problems, including depression, panic or general anxiety, compulsive behaviors, premen-strual mood or anxiety symptoms, bulimia, post-traumatic stress disor-der, insomnia, and others. According to data from the U.S. Centers for Disease Control, the antidepressants have become the most prescribed of all medications—even more than medications for hypertension, pain, or heart disease.[23] And this trend is perhaps most striking among young people. An article in *Psychology Today* noted, "The number-one prescribed drug for college students is not the birth control pill or an acne medication. It's Prozac. In second place are anti-anxiety agents. The number-three spot goes to all other anti-depressant SSRIs com-bined."[24]

It has taken a few years, but the bloom is fading from the SSRIs. Like every class of psychotropic drug before it, they have gradually shown that they are not without their problems. Though not gener-ally thought of as addictive, they often lose their effectiveness over time, and there is an unpleasant withdrawal syndrome when they are stopped after long-term use.

In the last few years, we have seen emerging controversies about the SSRIs. They have been associated with suicidal behavior, espe-cially in young people.[25] They have been linked with the rise in obesity and diabetes, and recently with bone weakening in older adults.[26] And now ecologists are concerned because these drugs, though diluted, are being found in our waterways (and the fish in them) and even drinking water, to unknown effect.

I am not against medication. There is a role for it, and I often prescribe it when I think it will be safe and helpful. But too often it does not remain helpful over the long term, and may even cause some of the very problems it is meant to relieve. There are chronic side effects to the SSRIs—such as weight gain, fatigue, loss of sexual interest, and mental or emotional dullness—that are often confused with the depression they are meant to treat. Others experience heightened anxiety or agitation, physical restlessness, muscle tension, or insomnia, all of which mimic an anxiety disorder.

If someone is suffering from an acute episode of anxiety or depression, I believe that every available measure should be taken to relieve the symptoms and help return the person to a healthier state. Often medications offer the fastest, most potent means to get relief. But they should be used judiciously. The mistake we too often make, in my opinion, is to rely too much on medications for the relief they give without thinking longer term.

What will lead to full recovery? What will prevent the condition from returning? And what will raise your overall level of resilience so that you can flow with future stresses without sinking into an illness? Despite the promise seemingly offered by each new medicine, history suggests that we look elsewhere for the most effective and lasting relief. And when it comes to really thriving, living fully and deeply, we are much better off looking for solutions from within.

The Roots of Resilience

How to Understand the Seven Types of Anxiety

IN MY first book, *The Chemistry of Joy*, I used an image of a water-cooler to describe my notion of resilience. Imagine that each of us has a similar vessel in our brain. In that container is an elixir that keeps us resilient and able to handle the stresses we face without developing symptoms or illness. It helps keep us vital and alive. The elixir gets used up as we face daily trials and expend our energy in the business of life.

Each person has a different-sized container, depending in large part on genetics, along with influences from our environment, the quality of caregiving that we received when young, and our temperament. But no matter how large or small the vessel, if we keep it adequately filled, we will remain energized, vital, and relatively free of symptoms.

This metaphor works well in part because it is hopeful yet real at the same time. It acknowledges that we are endowed with differing degrees of natural resilience—clearly some of us have greater tolerance for stress than others. But resilience can be used up. We can become depleted. No matter how great our capacity, there is a limit to how much stress we can withstand before breaking down in some way. Even the strongest among us will succumb if exposed to great enough strain for long enough periods of time. So to the extent that we are able, we must limit the amount of unhealthy stress to which we are exposed.

This metaphor is also empowering because it points out that there is a great deal that we can do to influence our capacity for resilience. Good self-care helps keep our containers filled in two ways. First, by being honest and aware of what is draining our reserves, we can look for ways to stop, or at least slow down, the loss of this precious elixir. Second, we can take measures to restore ourselves, to refill the container. We do this by giving the brain what it needs to produce a balanced array of chemical messengers, by giving the body what it needs to remain healthy and energized, and by giving the soul what it needs to live a rich and meaningful life.

But the metaphor of the watercooler is also insufficient. It doesn't describe our full human capacity for growth or change. Yes, it is crucial for us to honor the body and brain, and to do everything within our power to care for our physical selves. But it takes a lot of individual effort to be so diligent about self-care. And still we are left with our same relatively small container, striving to keep it filled, to keep ourselves afloat.

We need to have a larger view of ourselves, to be able to see beyond the limited personal scope that consumes so much of our consciousness. That is the stuff of transformation, and it involves turning toward the inner life of deep meaning and opening to the outer life of deep connection. It requires some sort of centering or contemplative practice. And it really is the task of a lifetime. This may sound daunting, but the rewards are great. It allows us to tap into a reservoir of resilience that is so much greater than any container we can possibly create on our own.

In this chapter, I'll first define the problem—I'll introduce you to the seven most common faces of anxiety. You'll probably recognize yourself in one (or several) of these types. In fact, as we've discussed, our brains are actually hardwired for many of these behaviors. But there is good news. Resilience, I have found, is also programmed into our brains. Once we understand how these natural self-preservation instincts have gone into overdrive and created anxiety, we'll then be able to correct the problem and restore our natural balance of happiness and resilience.

What's Gone Wrong?

I believe that it is our nature to be resilient. We have innate balance, strength, and wisdom that are our natural set point, and we return to it when allowed to do so. One way to think of resilience is having the ability to return to a state of health and well-being once we've been relieved of a stress or after a trouble has passed. Unfortunately, there are many things that can disrupt that state and create a sense of imbalance or disease.

Sometimes we feel fragile and easily thrown off course or out of alignment. Our resilience seems low. Other times we experience something that is so hard or lasts so long that we seem to lose our inborn resilience altogether. I hope you can believe me when I say that it is still there, waiting to be dusted off and recovered. But before doing that, it may be helpful to better understand the nature of the disruption, to be able to see more clearly what has gone wrong.

As a Western-trained psychiatrist, I have learned to think in terms of particular diagnoses, those that are described in the Diagnostic and Statistical Manual of Mental Disorders, known as the *DSM-IV*. The common anxiety disorders include such things as phobias, post-traumatic stress disorder, obsessive-compulsive disorder, panic disorder, and generalized anxiety disorder. If you read the *DSM-IV*, you will find that psychiatric diagnoses are made by using checklists of symptoms that correspond to the various labels.

There can be value in naming the condition, and the insurance system that we use requires that we do so. Yet many people dislike being labeled, while others can become rather attached to their diagnosis and begin to believe that is who they are. You may find relief in discovering that there is an illness called panic disorder, for example, that is causing your suffering. But that doesn't mean that you have to allow that term to become the way that you see yourself. It is just a condition that you have, rather than the person that you have become.

I'd like to consider the various faces of anxiety differently for a moment, thinking about how and where things have gone awry. Then perhaps we can see these conditions as the temporary errors that they are, and we can begin to understand how to put things right again.

Activating the Fear Circuit

When we left Jessica in chapter 2, she was lying in her bed at the end of the day of her car accident. She had been wisely vigilant while driving in the snow, had reacted quickly and efficiently to protect her children, and had shown appropriate concern for the other driver injured in the accident. Everything had gone as best it could, and no one was seriously hurt. But as she played the incident over and over in her mind, she kept ruminating about the other man in the accident: *What if he dies?* It was a thought that she could not let go, and what happened next shows the power of the mind to create anxiety.

The thought began to gradually consume her. Within a short time she had trouble driving a car, and it wasn't much longer before she felt afraid even being in a car with others driving. Later she couldn't even walk across a road without becoming fearful. She had a brief reprieve that spring and summer when the snow melted and the weather improved.

But the next winter her fears returned with a vengeance. By the time I saw her in January, she could not even drive one mile to the grocery store. She had frequent panic feelings which she described like this: "I go into a deep worry—it's *really* extreme. I feel that something really bad did happen, or that it could happen. I have a deep feeling of guilt."

Sometimes she would become tearful, start sweating, and feel that it was hard to breathe. Her heart would race, she would feel sick to her stomach, and her body would shake. She was unable to sleep, and spent her nights tossing and turning.

Over time she developed several compulsions. She had to check things such as her curling iron more than ten times to make sure she had unplugged it. She would return several times after leaving her home to be sure that the door was locked. "It gets really time-consuming," she said, and she had to plan her day with extra allowances for these rituals in order to get to work or pick up her kids on time.

Fear had seeped into every area of her life, and she was feeling pretty hopeless that it would ever improve—she had already been in therapy and on medication for months and things were not getting better. In fact, she wondered if the antidepressant medication was actually making her feel worse, because when she accidentally missed a dose, it seemed that her anxiety was a little less intense.

Despite all of this, she was not depressed. "I've come to accept it," she said—further testament to her strength. But of course she was hoping for relief, and was willing to do anything she could to get it. She was an ideal candidate for the Resilience Training Program, which helped her get off her medication and free herself from the spiral of anxiety. To help understand why this comprehensive approach works so well for someone like Jessica, let's first take a closer look at the parts of the brain that become affected if fear spreads into all areas of one's being.

I think of the circuit of fear as having three layers:

1. **The lower brain, which I refer to as "the reactive brain."** It receives input from the senses and reacts automatically if there is an immediate threat.
2. **The midbrain, which I call "the emotional brain."** This is where the emotions of fear and panic are generated, providing important signals that further decisions or actions are needed to respond to some perceived danger.
3. **The higher brain, or "the thinking brain."** This is where all the incoming information is considered and decisions can be made as to what response is needed, if any.

While each of the brain areas has a different function, the real key to understanding how the brain works is to remember the importance of communication and the flow of information.

The various parts of the brain are highly networked with one another, and they are communicating constantly. Information may flow from the bottom up, taking all the information from the sense organs, muscles, and autonomic nervous system and relaying it up from the lower parts of the brain to the upper levels, where it can be more thoroughly processed. Communication may also flow from the top down, so that the thinking part of the brain may, after reflection, have important memories, plans, or insights to pass along to the emotion centers or to the rest of the body for action. And then there are the key structures in the middle, the centers for emotion and memory, which serve as gateways, relay stations, alarm centers, and more.

Different patterns of anxiety may emerge depending upon where in this communication system things are off-kilter. Some problems occur because of underactivity or blockage, while other problems occur due to overly active areas or ineffective gateways that are letting too much information through.

The Seven Faces of Anxiety

DIRECTION OF FLOW	TYPE OF ANXIETY	KEY FEATURES
Bottom-up	Scarcity	Grasping, hoarding, wanting more: "There is not enough."
	Avoidance	Denial, avoiding things that seem risky: "That feels too scary."
Top-down	Worry	Overthinking, fear of future: "Something bad *may* happen."
	Learned fear	Caught in memory, fear of past: "Something bad *did* happen."
Muddled middle	Panic	Intense, overreactive fear: "Something horrible *is* happening."
	Rumination	Unhealthy, repetitive thoughts: "I can't stop thinking this way."
	Compulsivity	Unhealthy, repetitive behaviors: "I can't stop acting this way."

Bottom-Up Anxiety: Overly Vigilant

The types of anxiety that I associate with this level are what I refer to as *scarcity* and *avoidance*. Both have to do with being overly vigilant, seeing scarcity or danger where they don't exist. There is either an error in perception or a misreading of what one accurately perceives.

The lower parts of the brain are involved with some of our more basic survival needs, such as securing food, avoiding things that are dangerous, and fostering a sense of rhythm and ritual. It is the entry point for the sensory signals from the rest of the body, making it an ideal location for sensing danger and setting a tone for the rest of the brain's fear circuitry.

Scarcity refers to a sense that there is not enough. At the level of our most basic needs, that may mean that there is not enough food, drink, or even shelter or other forms of safety. This perception triggers intensely strong reactions to search for, grasp on to, and hoard what is needed. If someone is truly hungry or has inadequate shelter, then having such a reaction is not anxiety: it is a normal, built-in survival mechanism. Human beings who have the will to live will do nearly anything within their power to secure enough of what they need to survive.

But for most people with anxiety it is not a true need; it is just an inaccurate perception that there is a lack of food or something else that they desire. And the object of desire runs a wide gamut in our society. It can include anything that we crave or consume: sweets, alcohol, clothing, nicer cars, bigger homes, the latest gadgets, better jobs, more friends, more sex. These are just a few examples.

In a sense, the thing that we crave and grasp is not relevant. The experience can be the same, regardless of what it is that we desire. It begins with a thought, of which one is most likely unaware: *There is not enough* or *I am not enough*. There is a feeling of insufficiency. Then there tends to be a sense of tightening up, almost literally as if we are clinging to something. Tension builds and there may be a compulsive need to get whatever we've focused upon. Getting it relieves the tension, but only briefly, and then the desire returns and the cycle repeats itself, over and over. We are never truly satisfied.

Avoidance is nearly the opposite experience. Rather than craving, there is an aversion to something. Many phobias fall into this category, and some of them seem to be built-in or hardwired means of assisting our survival. Fears of snakes, spiders, or heights, for example, have obvious survival implications, but the reaction to them goes way overboard for some people. Then it is the reaction itself rather than the object of fear, which creates the problem.

One of the most common and troublesome types of avoidance has to do with social anxiety, sometimes referred to as "social phobia." Closely related to this is performance anxiety—the fear of public speaking or being onstage. These are problematic in part because they can't entirely be avoided, and in fact most people with avoidant anxiety really want to be able to connect more with other people, speak up in class, or speak or perform in public. But the fear of somehow being singled out, of becoming the center of unwanted attention, can be so strong that it seems impossible to do so. It is perhaps harder to see this as related to survival, but in some individuals it can be perceived as such a threat that these people may feel as if their very life is at stake. Jessica developed phobic avoidance, first to driving, then to riding in a car, and then to being near cars.

Again, it makes little difference whether survival is at issue or not, because the perception exists that it is. We misread cues or overinterpret what is going on, so the brain is tricked into thinking there is a real, even extreme threat. This experience also begins with a thought, usually unconscious, that this thing before us is truly frightening, and so it is. The experience that follows is one of pure fear, possibly to the point of panic.

In both of the bottom-up types of anxiety, the problem is that the brain is giving too much power to the lower centers. It is their job to be vigilant, to gather enough of the stuff for survival and to detect danger in the environment. But they are doing this too well, in a sense, and are not being tempered by the higher parts of the brain. It is not that we are thinking too much—we are not thinking enough. We are just perceiving and reacting.

There are physical approaches to calming this reaction, which we will explore in the next few chapters, but one of the most effective remedies for this is to shift the flow of communication from bottom up to top down. That is, we want to engage the thinking part of the brain in helpful ways: to see craving for what it is, to reassure ourselves that there is actually enough, to challenge the misperception that something is threatening when it is not, and to tell the vigilance centers that they can tone it down. We want to break through unconscious denial with gentle, conscious awareness. That is the practice of mindfulness, which will be described more fully in Part Two.

Top-Down Anxiety: Thinking Too Much

Whereas bottom-up anxiety involves thinking too little, in top-down anxiety we are thinking too much but don't see that we are doing so. Both worry and learned fear become reinforced by thinking in the same patterns over and over again. It is as if we are rehearsing, perfecting our fearful thoughts or fear-based memories through repeated practice. This is exactly what started the reign of terror in Jessica's life. She could not stop thinking about the accident and all the things that *could* have gone wrong but didn't.

It is our capacity to think as we do that sets humans apart from all other creatures. The prefrontal cortex is involved with the highest level of thought regarding our fears. It makes the final decision about what is a real threat and what isn't, sorts out memories to decide if they are relevant or not, and sets the emotional tone for the rest of the brain. We do not want to let this thinking mind, with all its power, run amok. If it is unleashed and that power is directed toward creating fearful anticipation or rehearsing fearful memories, they will fill our consciousness and the rest of the brain and body will fall into step. Fear can spread so much that we can quickly become consumed by it, as Jessica found out.

Worry is familiar to all of us—everyone is captured by it from time to time. But we don't want it to become a way of life. If we turn our thinking mind toward looking for what is wrong or what might go wrong, it will certainly find things to worry about—*plenty* of things. There are always conditions in our present environment that could become a threat, or situations that might come to pass that are frightening.

Seeing all the potential threats is not necessarily a problem. That is an important survival mechanism, and back when the threats to our survival were more obvious there may have been some genetic advantage favoring those who were better at it. The problem occurs when we scan for danger over and over again in the absence of any real threat. Though this area of the brain is associated with consciousness, when we engage in unhealthy worry we are doing so quite unconsciously. There is no way that we would intentionally create such a miserable state for ourselves. We don't realize that we are doing it, and we don't know how to break out of it.

Learned fear, also called *conditioned fear*, is another example of an important survival skill gone awry. In this case, the focus is on the past, although many people fear that they may experience a similar traumatic event in the future. I include past trauma (including PTSD) in this category, and some types of avoidance as well. For example, Jessica began to avoid driving out of an unconscious fear that she would have another accident. In another example, an Iraq war veteran may have witnessed an explosive device destroy the vehicle in front of him. A sound, smell, or sight that had nothing to do with the explosion may nonetheless have been part of that experience, so he is now conditioned to panic when he encounters a similar sound, smell, or sight in the future.

Likewise, many people who develop a fear of public speaking have actually had a bad experience with it in the past. They may have become anxious and their heart pounded; they blushed, became unfocused, and forgot what they were going to say. If that was not successfully processed, they may have become conditioned to react in a similar way at the very thought of having to speak in front of others in the future.

It is crucial for our survival to learn from experience so that if we have encountered something dangerous in the past, we can remember the signs and avoid it in the future. Normally the experience of fear itself subsides after the encounter, and we can let down our guard. We can rest assured that the fear response will be reactivated and warn us if we need it.

The problem for so many who have had bad experiences is that the fear reaction does not subside. Sometimes that is because we remain in a threatening environment, and if so, that must be dealt with. Often, though, the feelings of stress and fear are kept alive by rehearsing the memories, playing them like a video clip over and over again in the mind. The feelings can be as intense as they were in the actual situation.

It is the thinking brain that is supposed to direct our use of memory and decide how to anticipate the future. In both worry and learned fear, the thinking brain has lost its bearings and become part of the problem. Thinking too much, when it is done without guidance from a higher level of awareness, can be harmful to our health. With time and assistance, it is possible to rein in our overactive mind by consciously reclaiming the process of thinking and by learning to allow the mind to calm itself down.

Meanwhile, it can be helpful to intentionally change the direction of flow, going from top down to bottom up. For instance, you can learn to ground yourself in the body, to pay more attention to touch, sound, or the feel of your breath as you allow it to gradually deepen and slow. Giving the thinking mind something concrete to focus upon can disrupt its busy creation of fear.

In a recent study from the University of Oxford, for example, subjects who had just viewed trauma on film were less likely to develop flashbacks if they played the video game Tetris half an hour after seeing the trauma. The theory is that doing something that occupies the visual-spatial area of the brain does not allow it to consolidate those visual memories.[1] It pays to be intentional about where we place our thoughts.

The Muddled Middle: Stuck in a Circular Rut

This third and final category, which includes panic anxiety, rumination, and compulsivity, involves the important middle area of the brain, the area of emotion. This includes the limbic system and a few key structures around it. A relatively small area of the brain, this is where much of the scientific focus has been for the field of psychiatry, as well as the drug industry, as they seek remedies for emotional conditions.

The problems that occur here have less to do with direction of the flow of information. Instead, there is a disruption of that flow. Something has gone amiss in the communication between the brain areas, so that part of the circuit gets locked into the on position and becomes unable to shut itself down properly.

That occurs most clearly with *panic anxiety*, where the amygdala, the brain's "panic button," begins doing its job, but then can't stop doing it. The very feelings that occur during a panic attack, the sense that something really dire is about to happen, are completely normal when something dire *is* about to happen—as when Jessica was about to have her accident. Then we *should* feel alarmed, and that feeling lets us know that we have to take some protective action. But panic anxiety is like having a home alarm that is set to be too sensitive—it starts going off when there is very little threat, like Jessica driving to the grocery store, or even no threat at all.

Closely related to the amygdala is the hippocampus, the seat of memory. It becomes engaged when the panic button goes off, and it, too, can be overly activated, linking innocent situations with perceived threat. With prolonged stress and anxiety, the hippocampus can become impaired in its ability to store and retrieve memory. Cortisol, the long-acting stress hormone, can even cause the hippocampus to shrink.

I believe that most of the effects of long-term stress are reversible. If we can shut down the stress response and let the brain settle, all of these structures can return to their normal, healthy roles.

Rumination is also associated with something being "stuck" in the brain. In this case, it is a stuck pattern of thinking, a particular thought that goes round and round like a turning wheel—as when Jessica lay in her bed unable to stop thinking about the elderly man who was injured. This may sound a lot like worry, and indeed worry can take on a ruminative quality. But worry involves the creation of new thoughts, looking for new dangers, new things to anticipate with fear. There is nothing new when one ruminates. Animals classified as ruminants, including cattle, got this name because they chew their cud, going back over the same food again and again to aid in its digestion. Likewise, we keep chewing on the same few thoughts over and over again, as if doing so might help us digest them.

This ruminative pattern of thinking seems to be related to a problem with the cingulate cortex, which sits between the higher, prefrontal cortex and the areas of emotion below. The cingulate is supposed to aid in communication between them, and to help resolve conflict when that exists between the rational, thinking mind and the centers of emotion. When it becomes locked in the on position, we may think really, really hard about a dilemma, but that thinking is ineffective. We perseverate instead, and cannot resolve the conflict or make decisions.

This is a good example of how unproductive it can be to try to resolve internal conflicts through sheer effort. Our brain is working very hard. Yet the best thing we can do in this circumstance is to stop trying so hard—to allow the brain to settle, the effort to dissipate, the mind to clear. With a clear mind, the next decision or action to take usually becomes clear.

Compulsivity includes any kinds of behavior that we cannot stop doing, and in which there is a feeling of unpleasant tension that grows until we perform the action. Then the tension is released, at least partially, only to grow again until the behavior is repeated. There is an unending circuit of tension and release. As fear took over more and more of her brain, Jessica developed compulsive behaviors—checking her curling iron or the locks on the door.

With compulsivity, there seems to be a problem with the basal ganglia, a lower brain area associated with movement but also with monitoring and controlling the inflow of bottom-up communication. A gateway that should allow sensory input into the brain in a measured way can become ineffective, opening the floodgates and allowing information to overwhelm the system, creating unchecked loops of anxiety.

It may be because the basal ganglia assist with movement that some signs of compulsivity have to do with movement. Tics, nail biting, picking at the skin, or hair pulling are examples.

The basal ganglia are associated with dopamine, a neurotransmitter important for movement but also for the feelings of reward and pleasure. I believe that dopamine deficiencies can be connected to other compulsive problems, including those having to do with food, sex, gambling, and some drugs.

One type of compulsive behavior involves rituals, such as those seen in OCD (e.g., checking to see that a door is locked, hand washing, cleaning). Sometimes these behaviors (and other aspects of compulsivity) respond to drugs that increase the amount of serotonin in the brain, so measures that improve serotonin function can also be helpful. In Jessica's case, the drugs weren't helpful, but natural therapies were. We will explore natural means of supporting serotonin and calming the brain in the next few chapters.

What's *Not* Wrong? Resilience Is Our Nature

Western medicine is effective at dealing with illness but not as good at helping people achieve and maintain wellness. When disease is so clearly the focus, how could we expect it to be otherwise?

Most physicians see it as their job to find out what's wrong (diagnose the condition) and then try to fix it (prescribe a treatment). That is the role that we have been assigned, and one that we have accepted. But it is a vastly different thing to work at fixing problems than it is to help people live so full, vital, and balanced a life that the disease is unlikely to return.

Likewise, many patients become so focused upon what's wrong with them that they lose sight of what is *right*. They forget that they have strengths, remain essentially healthy, or at least have pockets of health that could be activated in their quest to relieve their suffering. When I first saw her, Jessica had lost sight of her basic goodness and underlying resilience, even though it was so apparent to everyone else.

We give power to that which we give attention, so that if we only see the unhealthy part of ourselves, that becomes enlarged out of proportion to how we really are. It is important to see very clearly what is wrong, but not to allow that view to take over. We must place more of our focus on what is *not* wrong with ourselves, seeing and claiming the resilience that is our nature. Focus upon that and see what grows.

The Seven Roots of Resilience

ASPECT OF RESILIENCE	AREA OF FOCUS	CORE PRACTICES
Balancing brain chemistry	Biochemical body	Diet, supplements, medications when needed
Managing energy	Energy body	Exercise, supplements, activities
Aligning with nature	Rhythmic body	Sleep, hormones, cycles of activity/rest, balanced lifestyle
Quieting the mind	Thinking mind	Mindfulness of breath, body, thought, speech
Skillfully facing emotions	Emotional mind	Awareness of inner experience, grounding in the moment, releasing "my story"
Cultivating a good heart	Heart capable of love	Opening to self-acceptance, loving-kindness, generosity, gratitude
Creating deep connections	Soul capable of unity	Connecting, developing a sense of belonging, seeing interconnection, knowing all will be well

The above chart summarizes my concept of resilience, which is really my understanding of who we are as whole human beings. These seven Roots of Resilience reflect different facets of the whole. The first three focus upon our physical selves, the body and what it requires to function as it is meant to. They provide the foundation for resilience, like the three legs of a stool, providing a stable platform for cultivating the rest of one's self. The three areas are interconnected, of course. If you improve your diet, for example, you will not only improve your brain chemistry but also have more energy. And if you exercise, you are also likely to sleep better, and so on.

The final four roots are reflections of the mind and soul, which constitute our inner selves. The fourth and fifth factors deal with thoughts and emotions—different aspects of the mind. Unhealthy thoughts and feelings are the source of much of our distress. The focus here is on learning to allow less harm to ourselves by either being unconscious of our thoughts and feelings or reacting to them in a way that makes things worse. Becoming more conscious of what we are thinking and feeling and more skilled at calming the mind and facing the emotions allows us to release ourselves from their grip. It is possible to step away from much of the distress that they cause.

The sixth and seventh roots, cultivating a good heart and creating deep connections, take us beyond our attempts to feel better. The focus here is upon developing positive, healthy inner qualities that build upon strengths that we already possess. They open us to the life we are longing for, where we feel more alive and engaged, more and more like the self we would wish to be. It feels so much better to live like this that it leaves little room for unhealthy fear, stress, or anxiety.

The Resilience Training Program that I will describe to you allows for all of these possibilities. This is a holistic model that offers a broad palette of options because there is more power in using a coherent and cohesive approach. You are in charge of this process, and you don't have to do everything all at once. You may never need to use all of these tools and skills. For example, you may feel so well just by balancing your brain chemistry or improving your energy that you may not feel a need to do more. Or perhaps you are already doing very well on the physical level, and it is the inner life that wants more attention.

The program is laid out in a series of steps that you can adapt to fit your own needs. Some you may easily begin right away, whereas others you may institute over time. You can keep refining your own program, as seems right to you. You can take the first step right now by believing that you can grow in your capacity to handle whatever is before you, no matter how stressful. More than that, know that you can live your life with greater fullness, vitality, and serenity, even when life is challenging.

4

Step 1:
Balance Your Brain Chemistry

How to Feed Your Brain for Optimal Mental Health

Let food be your medicine and medicine be your food.

—HIPPOCRATES

Key Points
- Eating better will always improve your health, including the health of the brain. It is inexpensive and risk-free.
- Your own health can only be as good as the health of your food sources, and that includes the entire food chain.
- The best source of healthy nutrients is a varied diet of whole foods that are mostly vegetables, grains, and fruits, with limited amounts of animal protein.
- It is through diet and nutrition that we have the best chance to affect gene expression. It is possible to turn off illness genes by changing the way we eat.

MANY PEOPLE today are understandably frustrated by the complicated and often conflicting information that they encounter about diet. It is good to remember that eating well is really not so hard to do. A hundred years ago, before there was much of a food industry, most people had pretty healthy diets. They ate whole foods that were in season, and they got their nutrients from a wider variety of foods than we do today. Food was minimally processed, so they had lots of fiber and other nutrients in their diets. They had ample vitamins and minerals, because the soils contained them. They got plenty of omega-3 fats from a variety of grains, eggs from healthy chickens, and meat from free-range farm animals or wild game. And no one had yet thought to put chemicals and other additives in food, so they weren't taking in a lot of things that the human body was never meant to have.

Today, eating well seems to have gotten a lot more complicated. Bringing clarity to nutrition is a challenge when so many experts seem to conflict with one another. The most clear and succinct advice regarding diet may be the phrase made famous by Michael Pollan, first in an essay for the *New York Times Magazine* and later in his book *In Defense of Food*: "Eat food. Not too much. Mostly plants."[1]

This simple statement makes it easier to sift through all the conflicting advice regarding diet and nutrition. First, eat whole, fresh food that has not been overly processed or filled with additives, just as people did until the last few decades. Second, don't eat too much—our bodies are not designed to take in as many calories as most of us do in our culture. There is growing scientific evidence suggesting that you can improve longevity and age-related memory by eating fewer calories (within reason, of course).[2] And third, there is a compelling argument that the healthiest diet is one that is mostly plant-based. Keep meat in your diet if you like, but use it as a side dish rather than the main course. Eat as many fresh, organic green vegetables as you can, along with fruits, root vegetables, whole grains, beans, and legumes.

In the Resilience Training Program, I am blessed to work with a gifted integrative nutritionist, Carolyn Denton, and much of what I know about nutrition I've learned by working together with her. Both she and I meet individually with every participant, to try to determine whether there are certain neurotransmitters that are missing, specific nutrients that may help correct a metabolic problem, or foods that the person is eating that may actually be aggravating his or her condition. We do not believe that everyone should eat the same diet, because we are all made a little differently, with different body types and different needs. Dietary needs may change over time, so at one point in your life you may feel best eating one way, and at a later point you may wish to eat differently.

Yet when we are dealing with anxiety or other stress-related symptoms, there are some straightforward approaches to diet that can help everyone. There are a few principles that I will share in this chapter that can help calm the brain and address the underlying problems that are promoting the brain chemical imbalance: things like inflammation or insulin sensitivity (which will be discussed further in chapter 6). Most of these suggestions will remain useful even after the anxiety has resolved or the period of stress has passed. Then, you may want to determine your own natural body-mind type and refine your diet to help keep you in balance. If you would like to learn more about this approach, refer to my earlier book, *The Chemistry of Joy*, which can help you decide what type you are and which diet is best for you to follow long-term.

Care and Feeding of Your Brain

Here are some core principles to help you regain your brain balance through diet, along with concrete steps to put those principles into practice:

PRINCIPLES FOR A RESILIENT DIET	PUTTING THEM INTO PRACTICE
1. Eat whole, natural foods.	Buy unprocessed, organic food as much as possible.
2. Eat a wider variety of foods.	Eat more seasonal, local foods. Discover new kinds of meats, vegetables, grains, nuts, and seeds.
3. Eat toxin-free (or at least less toxic) foods.	Avoid food with chemical additives. Be sure certain fruits and vegetables are organic. Buy hormone-free meat and dairy. Avoid certain seafood products.
4. Eat more brain-protective foods.	Look for colorful fruits and vegetables. Consume more omega-3 fats.
5. Eat more brain-nourishing foods.	Focus on complex carbohydrates. Eat modest amounts of lean protein. Get plenty of healthy, omega-3 fats.

Eat Whole, Natural Foods

Why would we eat anything other than real food? It is easy to understand, actually, because processed food is convenient and inexpensive, and it tastes good. Also, it comes packaged in increasingly appealing forms, and we are all susceptible to the power of advertising. When we are drawn to an interesting new product in the supermarket aisles, we aren't thinking, *Wait, we've evolved over thousands of years to eat natural, unprocessed foods—can my body really handle all the chemicals they've added to this? And don't I need a lot of the nutrients they've removed through processing?* We don't think that way, but we would feel better if we did.

This point was brought home to me recently when I toured a food museum. Breakfast cereals, introduced barely a hundred years ago, were originally intended to increase healthy eating options by processing grains to make them easier to prepare and eat, while still providing whole-grain nutrition. Next time you are in a grocery store, look at the breakfast cereal aisle, and you will have a good sense of what has happened in the past fifty years. The food industry has changed the way we grow, manufacture, and eat food. Cereals are increasingly more refined, have less fiber and more sugar, and contain more additives for flavor or to preserve the food longer on the shelf. It has not been to our advantage. Obesity, heart disease, insulin resistance and diabetes, and neurodegenerative diseases such as dementia, depression, and anxiety disorders—all the chronic illnesses related to the Western disease cluster—can be linked to these changes in the way we eat, along with our relative inactivity.[3]

Take Action

- There is a simple remedy to this. Try to reclaim eating in the way humans have always eaten prior to the past fifty years or so. As Michael Pollan suggests, "Don't eat anything your great-great-grandmother wouldn't have recognized as food."[4]
- You can still find foods that look more or less the same as

they always have, that are still in their original form. Shop at a food co-op, a natural foods store, or the natural foods section found in more and more supermarkets.

- Or follow the advice I heard years ago: stay along the perimeter of the store—in the produce aisle, the meat and dairy sections, the whole-grain breads—and avoid the central aisles where most of the packaged, processed foods reside.

Eat a Wider Variety of Food

It may surprise you that, despite the thousands of new food products being introduced to the market each year, our ancestors derived their nutrition from a much wider spectrum of food sources than we do today. That's because they had to—they didn't have year-round access to the same few foods, packaged in a dizzying array of different shapes and sizes that masquerade as variety.

For example, most of the meat-eaters in the United States today choose from one of three types of meat: beef, pork, or chicken. Most of these animals are raised in cramped conditions with little exercise and less than ideal diets, often supplemented with antibiotics and hormones to speed growth.

Contrast that with the more traditional human diet, where people ate less meat, but from a much greater variety of animals. Many of them were wild game that they hunted themselves, and others were domestic stock that roamed outdoors with plenty of exercise and a diet that was natural to them. Many cultures derived their protein mostly from seafood when the waters were still pure and chemical-free.

Another example of change in our diet is the monoculture of wheat, which provides the bulk of most people's calories. Previous generations ate many different types of grains, some of which are seldom

used today: barley, millet, buckwheat, spelt, and amaranth are examples. There used to be several different strains of wheat, which are
seldom cultivated today. We have become overreliant on a single grain
that for many people is the source of most of their daily calories. Think
about your own diet—do you ever go a day without eating some wheat
product? Even if you are trying to be healthy and eating whole-wheat
foods rather than refined white-flour bread, pasta, and baked goods, it
may still cause health problems to limit yourself to so few types of food.
You may be missing out on key nutrients that are found in one type of
grain but not another. Omega-3 fats are a good example—other grains
have a lot more of them than wheat.

A second, more complex problem is that many people eventually become intolerant to a food that they eat day in and day out, and
wheat is a common culprit. The Mayo Clinic and the University of
Minnesota just conducted a study in which they looked at this problem in an innovative way. They compared frozen blood samples taken
from Air Force recruits fifty years ago to blood samples taken from
both older and younger men living today. They found that wheat gluten intolerance (gluten sensitivity) has increased fourfold in that fifty-
year time frame, a jump that is far too high to be explained by genetics
alone. And the consequences can be serious—the condition increased
their risk of death fourfold.[5] The Mayo gastroenterologist who led the
study said of gluten intolerance, "It's become much more common. No
one knows why, but one reason might be rapid changes in eating habits and food processing over the last half-century."[6]

Take Action

- Eat foods as they are in season. Our diets are meant to
  change at different times of the year, which ensures that
  we get more variety in our diets, and also that we give

the body a break from the same old foods. If you go for a length of time without eating a certain food, your immune system may "forget" to react to it and you can lose your food sensitivity. Then you may be able to eat that food again, but not every day all year round.

- Shop at a local farmer's market, where you will likely find a wide variety of colorful, old-fashioned fruits and vegetables that are in season.
- Broaden your horizons by trying new foods that are unfamiliar to you. Especially pay attention to vegetables, grains, nuts, and seeds, and seek out as many as you can find. Try a variety of whole-grain breads, some of them with little or no wheat. Consider rye, millet, or rice breads. Spelt makes a good alternative to wheat. It is considered an ancient form of wheat but can often be eaten by people who have developed intolerance to wheat.
- And don't limit yourself to bread, which has by definition been partially processed. Look for grains that you have to cook for yourself, including millet, quinoa, oats, and brown rice.

Eat Toxin-free (or at Least Less Toxic) Foods

It may no longer be possible to completely eliminate toxins from your diet. They are everywhere. But if you really put your attention to it, you can vastly reduce your toxic exposure, and your brain will thank you for it.

A few things may seem obvious. First, if you are suffering from anxiety or insomnia or simply going through a period of stress, you should eliminate stimulants. That means coffee, caffeinated tea, and most soft drinks. Second, we should all minimize trans fats, found in most fried foods, baked goods, and many processed foods. Saturated fats, contained in meat, eggs, and dairy products, are also unhealthy if eaten in excess. It also stands to reason that eating fruits and vegetables laced with pesticides, milk and meat filled with hormones, and foods processed with chemical additives and artificial sweeteners might not be good for the brain's health.

Other toxins are more hidden. Many people, for example, have read that it is good to eat more fish, without realizing that they may expose themselves to heavy metals or other toxins by doing so. Since the earth's waterways are so polluted, and because toxins tend to become more concentrated as you go up the food chain, there are some fish that are unsafe to eat in even moderate quantities.

Take Action

- Take out the stimulants. While I don't consider caffeine to be a toxin for most people, it can be harmful when your brain is overactive. Until your symptoms resolve, eliminate it, or at least limit yourself to one or two beverages per day containing caffeine: coffee, black tea, or soda. I consider green tea to be mild enough that you may still be able to drink that, and it has so many other health benefits that it may be a good beverage option.

- Eliminate artificial sweeteners and high-fructose corn syrup. Despite the promise of guilt-free pleasure, there is no good reason to use artificial sweeteners. They do not help with weight loss and they may be neurotoxic. They should be avoided by anyone with anxiety or a sleep disturbance. Like caffeine, they can further aggravate an agitated mind. (Ironically, advertisers have caught on to the problems with artificial and high-fructose corn sweeteners, such as obesity and diabetes, and some are now hailing sugar as the "natural" choice for beverages. Sugar is the new health food.)

- Remember that many drugs can be stimulating: cold medicines (many contain decongestants), pain relievers (they may contain caffeine), and even some herbal remedies (especially those containing gotu kola or some forms of ginseng). Some people become stimulated by antidepressants or other psychiatric medications. Talk to your doctor if you feel *more* anxious or agitated after beginning or increasing any psychotropic medication.

- Reduce toxic fats: cut back on fried foods and baked goods. Limit your trips to fast-food restaurants. Most cooking oils, while not directly toxic, may throw the body out of balance when used in excess. Reduce your use of corn, safflower, canola, and sunflower oils.

- Do not buy most processed foods. This may require you to break some entrenched habits. Look at labels on the food you purchase. You don't have to understand all the terms listed in the ingredient list. In fact, if you can't understand them, and if there are a lot of long chemical names, you probably shouldn't eat it.

- Purchase meat and dairy products produced from animals that are free of growth hormones (look for milk labeled as "rBGH-free") and have not been exposed to large amounts of antibiotics. We should care about how the animals that we eat are raised. If their environment is healthy, with uncrowded conditions, nutritious food, and physical movement, they are less susceptible to disease and should not require antibiotics to keep them healthy. We are at the top of the food chain, and every link in that chain is important to our health. Any unhealthy element that is added lower down in that chain eventually works its way up to us.

- Get organically grown, pesticide-free produce as often as you can. If you can't afford to do so all the time, at least try to do so for those fruits and vegetables that are considered to have the highest pesticide levels. The box lists the latest recommendations from the Environmental Working Group:[7]

Highest in Pesticides: Buy These Organic

Peaches	Nectarines	Lettuce
Apples	Strawberries	Grapes
Bell peppers	Cherries	Carrots
Celery	Kale	Pears

Lowest in Pesticides: Buying Organic Is Less Important

Onions	Sweet peas	Broccoli
Avocados	Kiwis	Tomatoes
Sweet corn	Cabbage	Sweet potatoes
Pineapples	Eggplant	
Mangos	Papayas	
Asparagus	Watermelon	

- Choose seafood that gives you minimal exposure to contaminants. Generally speaking, the larger carnivorous fish can have the highest toxic load (for example, tuna, marlin, and swordfish). Even salmon, often recommended for its healthy omega-3 fats, is often contaminated due to poor salmon-farming practices. Wild Alaskan salmon is considered safer, as are smaller fish such as sardines or herring. The Environmental Working Group gives these suggestions for healthy seafood choices: "farmed catfish, mid-Atlantic blue crab, croaker, fish sticks (usually made from pollack), summer flounder, haddock, farmed trout, wild Pacific salmon, and shrimp."[8] The Environmental Defense Fund offers a Pocket Seafood Selector: Fish Choices That Are Good for You and the Ocean. This addresses not only choices that are healthy for you but also those that contribute to better fishing practices and a healthier ocean environment. You may download it free at www.edf.org/documents/1980_pocket_seafood_selector .pdf.

Eat More Brain-Protective Foods

We're not aware of it, but our bodies are constantly under siege at the cellular level as a result of our own metabolism. We convert the energy from our food into glucose and use that, along with oxygen, to fuel our bodies. The brain, small as it is, consumes a disproportionate amount of glucose. It is working all the time, after all, and even more so when we are feeling frightened or stressed. This process of metabolism, known as *oxidation*, leaves behind several by-products called *free radicals* that can be harmful if not cleaned up. The chemicals that perform that clean-up function are labeled *antioxidants*.

There are a few powerful antioxidant supplements that we will discuss later. Still, it's best to give the body what it needs through whole foods. The best source of antioxidant protection, by far, is to eat a wide variety of brightly colored fruits and vegetables daily. The phytonutrients that give color to these foods also provide health benefits. Scientists' attempts to divide out the separate constituents into supplements do not provide the same effects. This is a case where the whole is greater than the sum of its parts. You may still wish to take antioxidant supplements, but do not rely upon them entirely. Instead, let nature's wisdom provide what you need by eating a wide array of antioxidant-rich foods year-round. That was built into traditional diets—now we have to be more intentional.

Take Action

- Add color to your diet. Seek out brightly colored fruits and vegetables that cover the full spectrum: red, yellow, orange, blue, purple, and dark green.
- Eat foods that may help your body detoxify, especially the cruciferous vegetables, which are in the cabbage family (cabbage, broccoli, cauliflower, kale, collard greens, bok choy, broccoli rabe, Brussels sprouts).
- Boost your dietary sources of antioxidants. The box lists some of the foods highest in antioxidants, according to the United States Department of Agriculture.[9]

Beans: small red beans, pinto beans, red kidney beans, black beans
Fruits: blueberries, cranberries, blackberries, plums/prunes, raspberries, strawberries, cherries, apples
Vegetables: artichoke hearts, russet potatoes, dark leafy greens (e.g., kale, collard greens)
Nuts: pecans, walnuts, hazelnuts
Spices: cloves, cinnamon, oregano

Eat More Brain-Nourishing Foods

We are designed to process whole foods within our bodies, not to have them processed for us before we eat them. Yet that is exactly what has happened over the past fifty years as the food industry has found increasingly novel ways to take the "whole" out of foods and make them more and more refined. It began even earlier, with white flour and white rice. When the brown exterior is removed, grains are easier to digest (because much of the work has been done for us), taste better (because the remaining starchy inside is closer to sugar), and store more easily (because pests also find them less nourishing). But the processing also takes out nearly all of the fiber, vitamins, and other micronutrients, leaving basically pure carbohydrate. Our bodies still have to digest it and turn it into sugar, but it happens too quickly and easily for our own good.

The process is even faster with sugar and its high-powered cousin, high-fructose corn syrup. Admittedly, sugar tastes better than whole grains, and high-fructose corn syrup appeals to the taste buds more powerfully than whole corn products. But many of the problems we have with brain chemical imbalance occur because of the rapid and dramatic changes in our diets favoring these sources of empty calories, bereft of any real nutritional value.

High-fructose corn syrup, first introduced less than thirty years ago, has taken the food industry by storm, and has perhaps taken a toll on our nation's collective health as well. If you read food labels, you will find high-fructose corn syrup in most processed foods, carbonated sodas, candy, and even many fruit drinks. Over this period we have also seen a parallel rise in disorders of metabolism such as obesity and diabetes, especially among children and teens.[10]

Processed foods impact brain balance in several ways. If too many of our calories come from refined carbohydrates, we are more likely to become depleted of vitamins, minerals, and other micronutrients. The quick rise in blood sugar also triggers an equally fast release of serotonin from the neurons. This is why we often experience the brief high or soothing feelings that accompany a sugar binge. What many of us fail to recognize is that this boost is not only short-lived; it may also lead to further depletion of serotonin levels. Additionally, the rise in blood sugar over time leads to a condition called insulin resistance, causing a cascade of further damage. If you eat a diet rich in whole foods, you will eliminate many of the problems of blood sugar regulation.

Everyone needs carbohydrates, especially if you are suffering from the effects of anxiety, fear, or the stress response. Complex carbs are those carbohydrates that still have all their fiber and nutrients. They are "whole." Therefore, they provide just the right balance of fuel, slowly released, along with a host of vitamins and minerals that help the brain produce serotonin and the other key brain chemicals. The majority of your calories should come from the healthier whole carbohydrates.

Protein is the second major source of calories and nutrients. Proteins provide us with amino acids, the building blocks for the body's physical and chemical structure. Amino acids become hormones and neurotransmitters, allowing for communication between different areas of the brain and body. You need protein—but not as much as most people in Western countries consume.

In traditional diets, meat was eaten in small amounts, used as flavoring or perhaps to celebrate a special event. We have come to believe that meats are the only source of protein. In truth, the amino acids found in meats are present in vegetables as well. That's why herbivores such as cattle and horses can produce plenty of muscle and neurotransmitters without eating any meat.

How did we become such a meat-eating, high-protein society? As it became possible to raise animals with the efficiency of a modern factory, prices came down enough to make meat more widely accessible. Yet we pay a price for the convenience of modern factory farming. Consider the health implications from a diet with too many calories, too much saturated fat, and too much exposure to hormones, antibiotics, and other chemicals.

The sources of protein, like carbohydrates, are as important as the quantity. Animal proteins are more concentrated, break down more quickly, and cause a more rapid rise in amino acids. That favors production of the stimulating brain chemicals—not what you want when you're stressed.

Proteins sourced from vegetables, such as beans and legumes, in balance with complex carbs, provide a better combination for making the calming neurotransmitter serotonin. Serotonin production is enhanced by eating small amounts of protein several times a day while keeping your blood sugar stable by including a variety of complex carbohydrates. You do need *some* protein for serotonin production, because it requires the amino acid tryptophan. But tryptophan is best absorbed if it is not overshadowed by the other, more prevalent amino acids.

In an optimal diet you get your food from a variety of sources. Rely less on meat, especially red meat, as your primary protein source, and when you do eat meat, choose more grass-fed or free-range animal protein. Eat more seafood and more protein from vegetable sources: beans, legumes, whole grains, and even green vegetables provide good sources of protein.

The third source of calories is fat—one of the most confusing topics in nutrition. How do you choose healthy fats? How much and what type of fats are best for the brain? Are low-fat diets really necessary for weight loss or heart health?

For most people, very low-fat diets are not healthy. In fact, one of the best things you can do for your brain is to eat *more* omega-3 fats.

They are protective for the brain and also nourishing. They reduce inflammation and aid in glucose metabolism. They also get integrated into the neurons themselves, helping the nerve cells develop and function properly. They are especially important constituents of the cell membrane, helping it stay permeable, flexible, and able to receive the chemicals of communication, the neurotransmitters.

If you limit the unhealthy fats in your diet (trans and saturated fats), there is still an important distinction to make between omega-3 and omega-6 fats. The body needs both. A natural diet, like our ancestors ate, offered equal amounts of omega-3 and 6 fats. That's what our bodies evolved to use. But with the dietary changes described previously, that balance has been lost, and we now get twenty to thirty times more of the omega-6 fats than the omega-3s.[11] This imbalance is particularly hard on the brain, and also promotes the inflammatory response, which further affects brain function. The imbalance needs to be corrected by consciously adding more sources of omega-3 fats (olive oil, nuts, seeds, a variety of grains and vegetables, and seafood). You can also try to reduce sources of omega-6 by reducing your use of the common cooking oils soy, safflower, corn, peanut, and sunflower. Instead, use olive oil for low-heat cooking and grapeseed oil or organic expeller-pressed canola oil for high-heat cooking.

Take Action: Follow the Resilient Diet

- Eat more frequent meals and keep portions small. *Always* eat breakfast—after fasting overnight, your brain needs fresh fuel. Eat every four to five hours throughout the day to keep blood sugar steady.
- Ideally, eat three meals of 400–600 calories each, along with two or three snacks of 100–200 calories each. Have a snack in the late morning and midafternoon. You may also

want to add a small snack just before bedtime if you eat dinner early or wake at night feeling hungry.

- Have a modest amount of protein with each meal and snack (except at bedtime, when you may want to avoid protein).

- Ideally, consume approximately 60–70 grams of protein daily for women of average size and activity, and 90–100 grams for men. Increase this amount if you have larger muscle mass or regularly participate in more vigorous activity.

- Eat meat sparingly, especially red meat. Limit meat portions to 4–6 ounces, and no more than once daily, if possible. The size of your palm is a good way to estimate the amount of protein you need for a meal.

- Seek out other sources of protein, including eggs, dairy, beans and other legumes, vegetables, and a variety of protein powders (e.g., whey, rice, hemp, vegetable, and soy).

- Build your diet around whole, complex carbohydrates. Try to have some with each meal and snack.

- Your greatest volume of food should be from fresh, organic plants, especially leaves. They have most of the nutrient value (including healthy fats) with very few calories.

- Try to have at least two brightly colored foods on your plate at each meal, and include all the colors over the course of each week: green, yellow, red, orange, blue, and purple.

- Eat some kind of cruciferous vegetable every day. Choose from broccoli, kale, collard greens, cauliflower, Brussels sprouts, cabbage, bok choy, broccoli rabe, and broccolini.

- Include modest amounts of calorie-rich complex carbohydrates as well. Start with beans (red, black, pinto, kidney) and other legumes (lentils, split peas, peanuts). Next, choose from several different root vegetables (carrots, potatoes, sweet potatoes, yams, squash). Keep eating grains, but with slightly less frequency. Aim to rotate five to seven different whole grains, including rice, oats, quinoa, millet, amaranth, barley, corn, and wheat. Try not to eat any single grain every day—aim to eat wheat just two or three days per week, for example. Wheat and corn, because they are so prevalent, are also the grains to which you are more likely to develop food sensitivity.

- Include healthy fats with nearly every meal and snack.
- Make olive oil your primary oil. Use it for flavoring foods, as with dressings or marinades, and also for cooking at low to moderate heat.
- If you want a more neutral-flavored oil (e.g., for baking or for salad dressings), use walnut or flax oil.
- For high-heat cooking, use grapeseed or canola oil.
- Add a variety of nuts and seeds to your diet—they make especially good snacks along with fresh or dried fruits. Choose nuts such as walnuts, almonds, and cashews. Also, add more seeds to your diet, such as flax, hemp, and pumpkin. Since all nuts and seeds are high in fat content, don't eat large amounts. Just a small handful makes an ample snack.
- Eat fatty fish at least two or three times per week. Be sure to choose from the least toxic varieties listed previously. Cold-water fish are highest in omega-3s, and smaller fish (or those caught in less polluted waters) are safest—for example, wild Alaskan salmon, herring, and sardines.
- Stay well hydrated.
- Make pure water your main beverage. Begin each day

with two large glasses of water. Have another large glass between each meal and snack. You don't need a lot of fluid during mealtimes—it may dilute gastric enzymes. Don't drink much fluid in the evening.

- If you like green tea, you can drink it throughout the day. It does contain a small amount of caffeine, so stop early enough to protect your sleep.

- Limit fruit juices. You are better off eating the whole fruit—you need the fiber to balance the rich concentration of the fruit's sugar (fructose).

- Try drinks containing healthy bacteria, including kefir and some of the new fruit drinks that have added probiotics.

- Eat more slowly.

- Fast food is a symptom of our underlying lifestyle. Counter the urge to hurry and remain in stress mode by slowing down when you eat.

- Eating should be pleasurable. Food should taste good. To really enjoy it, you must take your time. When you really pay attention to the taste, texture, and quality of the food you are eating, you will naturally make better food choices. Quality food brings more pleasure than fast or processed food.

- You will also tend to eat less by eating slowly. When you are more present and have a fuller experience of your food, you derive more pleasure from less food. You also give your body time to register that it has had enough, so you can stop eating before becoming full.

- One of the traditional values associated with eating is gratitude. Take time to notice the bounty before you, the beauty of the food, its texture and flavor. Reflect for a moment on the source of your food: the soil, sunlight, and pure water that went into its growth; the many hands involved in growing, harvesting, and transporting it; the gift of its preparation for you; the restoring of your body that comes from eating healthy nutrients.

- Check out the Slow Food Movement. It is a grassroots effort to counter the fast-food lifestyle and to reclaim the beauty and pleasure of eating. "By reawakening and training their senses, Slow Food helps people rediscover the joys of eating and understand the importance of caring where their food comes from, who makes it and how it's made."[12] You can learn more at www.slowfood.com or www.slowfoodusa.org.

Someday you may be able to get dietary recommendations tailored specifically for your own genetic makeup. There is a burgeoning field known as *nutritional genomics* that promises to do just that.[13] Meanwhile, following the Resilient Diet will gently bring your body and your brain back into the healthy balance that is your natural state.

It takes time, so stay with it. Giving your brain what it needs through diet is the surest way to balance brain chemistry in the long run. Even so, there are times when you need more support. In the next chapter, we will explore natural means to calm the brain, correct brain chemical imbalances, and help you recover from the damaging effects of long-term stress.

Step 1 (Continued): Balance Your Brain Chemistry

How to Support Your Brain with Safe Nutritional Supplements

The desire to take medicine is perhaps the greatest feature which distinguishes man from animals.

—SIR WILLIAM OSLER

Key Points

- In order to work properly, the brain must have the right balance of chemicals called neurotransmitters. The only way it can produce them is for you to bring the necessary nutrients into your body.
- Nutritional supplements are not intended to replace whole foods. They are supplements to a healthy overall diet.
- When used properly, nutritional supplements and herbal therapies may help restore brain balance, soften the damaging effects of the stress response, and prevent the recurrence of illness.

MODERN PSYCHIATRY has become too narrowly focused upon brain chemistry and the myriad attempts to manipulate it with medications. This is unfortunate, because it reduces the suffering of human beings to too small a scale. We are so much more than serotonin and dopamine receptors. Yet we ignore brain chemistry, and the rest of the physical body, at our peril. We *are* more than our neurotransmitters. But we are *partly* our neurotransmitters, and if they remain imbalanced, you will not feel well for long.

Using medications to try to improve brain chemistry can offer relief, at least in the short term. But medications do not restore normal levels of neurotransmitters, nor even promote normal function. They manipulate the brain chemistry to achieve their desired effects.

SSRIs, for example, prevent the reuptake (or recycling) of serotonin from the space between the nerve cells (the synapse). This allows the chemical to remain in the area of activity for a longer period of time. And the benzodiazepines, such as Valium, Ativan, and Xanax, work by stimulating the GABA receptors, thus mimicking the calming effects of GABA in the brain.

With time the brain accommodates to medications and they often lose their effectiveness, requiring higher doses or different drugs. When you try to stop them, there are frequently withdrawal symptoms that feel worse than the original problem. And even if it seems to be working, it is a mistake to rely too much upon a medication and then ignore the rest of what makes us resilient.

If we want to restore resilience and prevent the recurrence of illness, then we must give the brain what it needs in order to do its job. That requires paying attention to what we take into our bodies. If we can understand what is required for normal function and what happens when it is missing, then perhaps we can restore balance as naturally as possible.

For instance, when the brain produces a neurotransmitter, it starts with a raw ingredient, usually an amino acid from the diet or another chemical that is already present in the brain. Enzymes are then used to convert the amino acid into the needed brain chemical. By understanding this process in detail, we can take measures to assure an ample supply of the raw ingredients and also enhance the activity of the enzymes. There are various cofactors, for example, that help the enzymes work faster (e.g., the B vitamins).

Understanding the function of nutrients allows for more subtle and natural interventions than standard medical practice, and if they are taken appropriately, I believe that they can work better and have fewer side effects than medication. The "toolbox" goes beyond supplements, of course, and includes diet, exercise, lifestyle changes, and body-mind practices such as meditation, all discussed elsewhere in this book. In this chapter we will focus on several different categories of supplements, including vitamins, minerals, amino acids, and herbs.

The Talking Brain

The neurotransmitters are chemicals that enable the different parts of the brain to stay in touch with one another and coordinate their roles. The table below summarizes the key players in the fear circuitry, what they do, and how to support them nutritionally. After describing them individually, we will consider the most useful supplements, and then I'll put it all together in the Resilient Supplement Plan.

BRAIN CHEMICAL	ROLE IN THE FEAR CIRCUITRY	NUTRITIONAL SUPPORT
Glutamate, the excitatory chemical	Heightens overall brain activity	Taurine, NAC, green tea, vitamin D_3, magnesium, omega-3s

GABA, the inhibitory chemical	Slows overall brain activity	GABA, L-theanine, taurine, vitamin B_6, zinc, inositol, herbal therapies
Norepinephrine, the arousal chemical	Raises level of alertness	L-theanine, NAC, omega-3s, inositol
Dopamine, the reward chemical	Focuses attention and enhances pleasure and reward	L-theanine, B vitamins, omega-3s, St. John's wort, ginkgo
Serotonin, the soothing chemical	Calms, regulates sleep and appetite, protects against stress	Tryptophan/5-HTP, DHEA, folic acid, vitamin B_6, vitamin B_{12}, vitamin D, omega-3s, St. John's wort
CRH/cortisol, the stress hormone	Prolonged elevation leads to fat storage, insulin resistance, degenerative brain disorders, memory loss, inflammation	DHEA, B vitamins, antioxidants, herbal adaptogens

Calm Yourself: Balance Glutamate and GABA

Our bodies are truly elegant in their design, and this is especially apparent with brain function. One common element of this design is a binary system, wherein one chemical activates a process while its partner turns it off again. That is true of the brain chemicals glutamate and GABA, which together account for over 80 percent of brain activity. Glutamate accelerates brain activity—it is excitatory. GABA, on the other hand, puts the brakes on brain activity—it is inhibitory. Together, they keep the brain humming along at just the right pace—not too fast, not too slow.

How Do You Know if Glutamate and GABA Are Imbalanced?

If you have developed any of the seven types of anxiety, then you know that your balance of these two chemicals has been thrown off and the brain's activity level is turned up too high, at least in some areas of the brain.

Remember that all of these chemicals are necessary and even beneficial when they are in balance and working properly. But it is possible to have too much glutamate for your own good. If it becomes truly excessive, then the overactivation that results can become outright dangerous to the cells. Glutamate then changes from being simply excitatory to becoming excitotoxic, and this may result in the premature death of the cell.[1] This process may be related to the later development of neurodegenerative diseases such as Alzheimer's or Parkinson's disease.[2] This is not a good state for your brain to be in for very long.

Additionally, your GABA levels may have fallen too low so that there is not enough inhibition to keep glutamate in check. Like a car that has lost its brake fluid, you may have lost the ability to slow things down. To remedy this imbalance, we can find ways to either reduce the effects of glutamate, enhance the activity of GABA, or both. Many of the measures we'll discuss have a positive effect on both.

The balancing supplements for glutamate and GABA include the amino acids taurine, GABA, and L-theanine; the antioxidants NAC and green tea; vitamins B_6 and D; the minerals magnesium and zinc; omega-3 fatty acids; and several herbal therapies. They are outlined in detail below.

Disarm Yourself: Reduce Norepinephrine

Norepinephrine raises our level of alertness and arousal, putting the amygdala on high alert to set off the alarms in case danger arises. That is well and good if you're doing something like hunting or evading capture, but not helpful if you are speaking in front of a group or if you have developed panic anxiety for any reason. With depression there is often too little norepinephrine, but in anxiety it is frequently elevated and needs to be toned down.

How Do You Know if Norepinephrine Is Excessive?

Norepinephrine is the brain's version of epinephrine, which also goes by the name adrenaline. Most of us have a vision of what happens when we're "running on adrenaline," and it is similar to the feeling you may have had from drinking too much caffeine, which also elevates norepinephrine's effects. Physically, there may be a rapid heart rate, shallow and rapid breathing, elevated blood pressure, cold extremities, muscle tension, and shakiness. At an emotional level, you may feel panicky, as if something awful is about to happen. And mentally, your mind may go blank as you find that you can't think clearly or remember things, no matter how hard you try.

You can tone down the effects of norepinephrine by taking the amino acid L-theanine, the antioxidant NAC, inositol, and the omega-3 fatty acids. You should also avoid caffeine.

Reward Yourself: Balance Dopamine

The effects of dopamine are more complex than those of norepinephrine, at least in regard to anxiety. In some ways, they have a similar function. Both tend to be energizing and aid in mental focus and concentration. Both can aggravate anxiety when levels are way too high. But dopamine has some beneficial effects against anxiety as well, such as improving motivation and the experience of pleasure. It also enhances microcirculation in parts of the brain.[3] Unless dopamine becomes really excessive, your anxiety may improve if you gently boost your dopamine levels.

How Do You Know if Dopamine Is Deficient?

Signs of dopamine deficiency include feeling apathetic and fatigued, difficulty losing weight, feeling unmotivated (as with exercise), low sex drive, and general difficulty getting pleasure from things. If you have these signs along with anxiety, consider taking these measures to boost dopamine function: B vitamins, omega-3 fatty acids, L-theanine, and herbal therapies such as ginkgo biloba and St. John's wort.

Soothe Yourself: Boost Serotonin

Nearly everyone feels better when their serotonin levels are optimal. It has such a wide array of functions, involved with everything from sleep to appetite to impulse control to sexual desire. It is the brain chemical that helps soothe us when we feel stressed or threatened, and it offers considerable protection to the brain against the damaging effects of cortisol.

Serotonin's broad benefits may explain why Prozac and the other SSRIs took the world by storm in the 1990s. It took a while for the shortcomings of these medications to become clear—problems such as agitation, numbing of emotions and sexual feelings, weight gain, insomnia, and fatigue. The SSRIs are *not* the panacea that they initially appeared to be, as we've seen. Yet the problem remains: millions of people are serotonin-depleted and suffer from the impacts of stress and anxiety (not to mention depression) as a result.

How Do You Know if Serotonin Is Deficient?

Because it is such a key brain chemical, the signs of serotonin depletion are many: insomnia (or irregular circadian rhythms); craving sweets and other carbohydrates; frequent muscle aches and pains; impulsive behaviors; moodiness, especially sadness, anxiety, and irritability; feeling emotionally sensitive or vulnerable; feeling insecure, lacking self-confidence; and low stress tolerance.

Most people with anxiety, especially if their mood is low as well, may benefit by boosting their serotonin levels. In addition to following the Resilient Diet, which is designed to help with serotonin production, consider taking the following supplements: the amino acid L-tryptophan or the related precursor 5-HTP, the hormone DHEA, the B vitamins and vitamin D, omega-3 fats, and the herb St. John's wort. It also helps to take measures to reduce inflammation (see chapter 6), which frees up a key metabolic pathway to produce more serotonin.[4]

Protect Yourself: Take the Sting out of Cortisol

Do you long for a stress-free life? Do you wish that your stress hormones would go away and not come back? Actually, you wouldn't want either of these, any more than you would want a life without pain. No one wants to be in pain all the time, but to be unable to feel pain at all creates a nightmare of its own. Likewise, if you were unable to mount a stress response, if your body suddenly became unable to produce the stress hormones, your physiology would collapse.

Stress is not the problem. It is *unremitting* stress and a constantly elevated level of cortisol that create the problems. The consequences can be severe. If it goes unchecked, elevated cortisol may cause weight gain, insulin resistance, or even type 2 diabetes; elevated blood pressure and coronary artery disease; memory problems and possibly dementia and other neurodegenerative diseases; and immune system problems, which may impair your body's ability to fend off diseases of all types, including autoimmune disorders and even cancers.[5]

The ultimate answer to this risk is to bring stress and the stress hormones back into a normal, healthy range. Still, we all go through highly stressful periods in our lives from time to time. If you have been overly stressed for months or years, it may take a long time to bring the stress response back into line. Meanwhile, it is crucial to protect yourself with the Resilient Diet and some of the following supplements: the steroid hormone DHEA, which tones down the effects of cortisol; the B vitamins, which help keep homocysteine (a harmful amino acid associated with heart disease, depression, and anxiety) in check; antioxidants; and herbal adaptogens such as rhodiola (see below).[6]

The Resilient Supplement Plan

The following table summarizes the supplements I recommend to support the brain and restore it to a more resilient state.

SUPPLEMENT	TYPICAL DOSAGE	COMMENTS
Multivitamin or B complex	As directed on bottle. Aim for 25 mg of B_6 twice daily as a rule of thumb.	If cost is a factor, you may choose a B complex.
Vitamin D_3 (vitamin D_3 is the easier form of vitamin D for the body to use)	2,000 IU from October through April. May reduce to 1,000 IU in summer, or stop if in the sun 15–20 minutes daily.	Consider getting your vitamin D level tested, especially if you live in the north and/or you have dark skin.
Omega-3: fish oil and/ or flaxseed	2,000–4,000 mg fish oil; may augment with 2 tablespoons ground flaxseed daily.	Fish oil is preferred, but vegetarians and the cost-conscious may use flaxseed.

Minerals: calcium, magnesium, zinc	Calcium citrate: 500–800 mg daily. Magnesium: 400–600 mg daily. Zinc: 15–30 mg daily.	Most men do not need calcium. Zinc may be best absorbed taken separately from other minerals.
Tonic herb: rhodiola	200 mg daily.	An herbal adaptogen, this may improve the body's general response to stress.
Therapeutic supplements: amino acids, hormones, medicinal herbs	Varies—see below.	Consider these like medication: talk to your doctor before taking these.

The first four categories of supplements listed are those that I consider to be the core foundational support for anyone dealing with stress-related problems such as anxiety. By themselves, they are unlikely to give dramatic relief. But if they are missing or deficient, it makes it much harder for other measures to be really helpful.

I've added a fifth supplement to the foundational program—rhodiola—that I consider optional. I include it among the core supplements because it can provide safe, long-term support for both mood and anxiety and has a broadly beneficial effect on the stress response system.

After we've covered the basic supplements, I will describe a handful of stronger, more medicinal natural therapies that can be added to your core supplement program if you need additional support. These include amino acids, hormones, and herbs.

The Foundational Supplements

Multivitamin or B Complex

Recently there have been reports suggesting that multivitamins are ineffective and a waste of money, an assertion that some doctors have always maintained. The most notable of these reports came from the Women's Health Initiative, a large population-based study observing more than 160,000 women over the long term. They found that nearly 42 percent of the women used multivitamins, which had no discernible effect on rates of cancer, heart disease, or mortality.[7]

These are strong findings, but it is a mistake to conclude from this that there is no value whatsoever in taking a multivitamin. It only tells us that the standard multivitamin taken by most women does not prevent cancer, heart disease, or other causes of death. I still believe that there is value in adding nutritional support in the form of a high-quality multivitamin, especially during periods of physical or emotional stress.

There is a huge disparity between nutritional supplements in terms of quality, and that is certainly true of multivitamins. Most of them are not very good and add so little benefit that they may indeed be a waste of money. The average multivitamin, for example, has very low doses of the B vitamins—the most important vitamins in terms of preventing the negative effects of stress. I prefer that my patients use a high-quality multivitamin if possible, because it will also contain a number of micronutrients and good antioxidant protection. But if it seems too expensive (they often cost about $30 per month), you may choose to forgo the multivitamin and just use a B complex. These typically cost only $8–10 per month.

Gene expression (whether or not a gene is active) can be affected by environmental factors, including diet. A process known as *methylation* helps to signal a gene sequence to turn on or off, thereby influencing whether or not a given disease is expressed. Vitamins B_6, B_{12}, and folate (also called folic acid) have a strongly positive influence on methylation, which can suppress the production of cortisol.[8] Methylation also reduces the harmful amino acid homocysteine.[9] Vitamin B_6 also aids in the production of both GABA and serotonin, the two brain chemicals most likely to calm the fires of anxiety.[10]

How Much of the B Vitamins Should You Take?

I recommend 25–100 mg daily of B_6 (in the form of pyridoxal-5-phosphate, or pyridoxine), 400–800 mg daily of folic acid, and 50–200 mcg daily of B_{12}. For the sake of simplicity, I often suggest to my patients that they look at the label to see how much B_6 their vitamin contains. If it is in the range that I recommend above, then the chances are that the other B vitamins will be sufficient as well.

B vitamins are used quickly, so it may be best to take half of the daily dose in the morning and the other half in the evening, with food. However, some people feel overly energized by B vitamins and may need to take it all in the morning, or even to reduce the dose to half of the above recommendation, in order to get good-quality sleep.

Note that as they age, many people do not absorb B_{12} effectively and may need higher doses, up to 500 mcg daily. To bypass this absorption problem, you may take it sublingually (under the tongue) or have your doctor administer a B_{12} injection.

One more word about folic acid. There are several steps required to turn dietary folate into the most activate form of folate, known by the name 5-MTHF (5-methyltetrahydrofolate). Some people don't convert folate very efficiently, due to differences in enzyme levels, and they may achieve a much stronger effect by using a product that is already activated. It is now available and can be found by looking for MTHF on the label.[11]

Vitamin D$_3$

In the past few years we have become much more aware of the importance of vitamin D. Once thought to be involved mostly with calcium metabolism and bone health, it is really a hormone rather than a vitamin and has a much wider array of effects than had been thought. It has been linked to everything from heart health to cancer prevention, from diabetes to chronic pain. Scientists have even begun to consider vitamin D deficiency as a possible cause of autism.[12]

Vitamin D plays a role in brain health, and low levels are thought to be one of the reasons for depression, especially among the elderly and those living in northern latitudes.[13] Vitamin D and serotonin receptors are closely linked in the brain, and vitamin D aids in the production of serotonin.[14] It also protects against the effects of stress. For example, if glutamate levels get too high, vitamin D offers protection to the nerve cells, reducing the risk of cell death.[15]

How Much Vitamin D Should You Get?

One of the amazing things we've learned about vitamin D is just how many people are deficient. In Minnesota, where I live, we have found that about 80 percent of our patients have low levels of vitamin D, even when we measured their levels at the end of the summer. Your body can produce vitamin D on its your own with sun exposure, but few people spend much time in the sun anymore, and when they do, they often protect their skin with sunscreen (a good idea for most people).

Even with lots of sun exposure, there is no guarantee that you will have adequate vitamin D levels. One study recently done in Hawaii, where participants spent an average of eleven hours per week outdoors (without sunscreen), found that half of them *still* had low levels of vitamin D.[16]

I recommend supplementing with at least 2,000 IU daily of vitamin D_3 (cholecalciferol) in the months from October through April, and continuing to take 1,000 IU daily in the summer, unless you get out in the sun regularly. You only need about fifteen minutes of sun exposure without sunscreen to get the maximum benefit from the sun.

Since there is so much individual variability in vitamin D levels, and even in the ability to produce it from sun exposure, I think it is a good idea to have your level checked by getting a serum 25-hydroxy vitamin D test. Your doctor can order it, and it is not expensive. It will allow for much more refined supplementation, and if you discover that your levels are extremely low, you may experience a dramatic improvement in all sorts of symptoms after levels are restored.

Omega-3s

Omega-3 fatty acids play a central role in healthy brain function, in part because nerve cell membranes are largely made of fat. The omega-3s stabilize the cell membranes, allowing them to be more flexible and permeable so that they let in the chemicals the cells need. They also play a role in the neurons' ability to communicate with one another, and have a general calming influence on the central nervous system.

Omega-3s have been studied extensively, particularly in treating depression and bipolar illness, and continue to show positive effects.[17] In addition, they reduce inflammation throughout the body, including the brain. Since there is such a strong connection between inflammation and the chronic stress response, I see every reason to boost omega-3 levels and very little risk. Caution should be used if you have a bleeding disorder or take anticoagulants (such as Coumadin), but otherwise this is considered a very safe supplement to take.

How Much Omega-3 Should You Take, and in What Form?

I believe that the most effective form of omega-3 comes from fish oil. It should contain both EPA and DHA, typically in about a 3:2 ratio. It is possible to get plenty of omega-3 fatty acids from non-fish sources, but not everyone can convert the form of omega-3 (known as ALA) found in those sources into the forms the brain needs (EPA and DHA). If you do take a fish oil supplement, be sure that it is of high quality. It should be molecularly distilled so that it does not contain any mercury or other toxins.

I recommend at least 2,000 mg daily of highly concentrated fish oil (or 4,000 mg if you have signs of inflammation or mood instability). This should give you approximately 600 mg of EPA and 400 mg of DHA per day. Store it in the refrigerator or freezer to reduce the unpleasant "fish burps."

For vegetarians, or those on a tighter budget, consider 2 tablespoons of ground flaxseed per day. Buy flax seeds whole and grind just enough for a week at a time (use a coffee grinder). Store it in the refrigerator. Hemp products (oil or seeds) are good vegetarian sources of omega-3s.

Minerals: Calcium, Magnesium, and Zinc

Calcium is important for proper nerve cell function and often helps sleep, though it is not a powerful sleep aid. Together with vitamin D, it is also crucial for bone health in women. In men there has been an association between higher calcium levels and the risk of prostate cancer, so I do not recommend that men take any additional calcium beyond what they get in their food.

Among the minerals, magnesium is king where stress and anxiety are concerned. Magnesium has long been known to be a relaxant, helpful to reduce muscle tension and anxiety and promote sleep. It also protects nerve cells from the excitotoxic effects of glutamate, aids in energy production within the cells, and helps with glucose metabolism.[18]

Zinc is heavily involved with the immune system, and low zinc levels are associated with inflammation. This combination of inflammation and zinc deficiency may make it harder to recover from stress-related illnesses.[19] The highest concentrations of zinc within the body are actually in the brain, and zinc is often located right next to the serotonin receptors. Scientists think that it may work to make serotonin more effective, and it also has a role in the balance of glutamate/GABA and even in neuroplasticity.[20]

How Should You Supplement Minerals?

If you are following the Resilient Diet and taking a good-quality multivatimin, most of your mineral needs should be covered, including zinc. But you may still need to add a supplement for calcium and magnesium. Here are the daily doses I recommend:

- *Calcium.* Women should take 500–800 mg as calcium citrate. With food sources, aim for approximately 1,200–1,500 mg total daily dose. Men do not need to take a calcium supplement, and can get by with 400–600 mg daily from food.
- *Magnesium.* The daily dose is 400–600 mg in the form of magnesium citrate, taurinate, succinate, or glycinate. Or if you have muscle soreness, you may want to use magnesium malate (also called magnesium with malic acid).
- *Zinc.* While many multivitamins give you zinc in a dose of 15–30 mg daily, you may need up to 50 mg or more if you have been found to be deficient through laboratory tests.

Zinc is often combined with calcium and magnesium but may be better absorbed if taken separately.

Tonic Herb: Rhodiola

A group of herbs known as *herbal adaptogens* or *tonic herbs* have long been used to strengthen immunity, improve energy, and enhance the body's ability to handle stress. Some of these may be familiar, such as ginseng or reishi mushrooms. My favorite for someone with stress, anxiety, or even depression is *Rhodiola rosea*, also known as arctic root.

Traditionally, rhodiola has been used to improve energy and mental focus, but recent studies have looked at its benefits with anxiety and depression.[21] A small study done at UCLA in 2008 showed that participants with general anxiety improved greatly on rhodiola, with minimal side effects.[22] It may work by improving serotonin and dopamine levels and counteracting the effects of cortisol.[23]

How Do You Take Rhodiola?

Look for an extract standardized to at least 3 percent rosavins and about 1 percent salidrosides. Take as directed on the label. A typical dosage is 100–250 mg twice daily, with breakfast and dinner. While it usually improves anxiety and even sleep, it is usually best not to take it just before bedtime. If it feels energizing, take it early in the day, with breakfast and lunch.

Rhodiola, like all the tonic herbs, is considered safe for long-term use and is not known to interact with medications.

The Therapeutic Supplements

In addition to the basic supplements, there are several therapeutic supplements, summarized in the table below.

SUPPLEMENT	TYPICAL DOSAGE	COMMENTS
L-theanine	100–200 mg twice daily.	Found in green tea; can be both calming and focusing.
5-HTP	50–100 mg up to three times daily.	Boosts serotonin. Helps anxiety and depression.
NAC	600 mg up to three or four times daily.	A potent antioxidant; recently shown to treat OCD.
Taurine	500 mg once or twice daily.	Improves glutamate/GABA function.
Inositol	500–1,000 mg two to three times daily (studies use 12–18 g per day).	Often considered a B vitamin, it can effectively treat panic, OCD, and phobic anxiety.
GABA	250–750 mg up to three times daily.	Does not cross easily into the brain, so other measures may have more effect on GABA.
DHEA	5–10 mg daily, up to 50 mg daily.	A hormone, it may increase risk of prostate or endometrial cancers. Check with your doctor and get levels tested before taking.
Therapeutic herbs (passionflower, valerian, St. John's wort, ginkgo)	Varies—see below.	

I consider these supplements to be medicinal, with stronger therapeutic effects than the basic supplements listed above. I've listed them roughly in the order in which I recommend them for the treatment of anxiety, with my first choices listed at the top. The exception to that is the category of "therapeutic herbs," which is at the end simply because there are several to be considered.

Some of these supplements can cause side effects, but most people tolerate them much better than prescription medications. They are generally considered safe. However, they should not be added to prescription medications without your doctor's knowledge and supervision.

If you are taking medication already, be sure to talk with your doctor before adding any of the supplements from these categories. And if you are considering going off medication, remember never to stop your medication suddenly—always consult with your doctor about how to safely taper off any psychiatric medication.

L-theanine

L-theanine is an amino acid found in high concentrations in green tea. But you would have to consume an awful lot of it to get a therapeutic dose of theanine. You can get more by taking a green tea extract, but you can also take a supplement containing L-theanine alone, or in combination with other calming agents.

One of the reasons I like L-theanine is because it works on so many neurotransmitters at once: it boosts GABA and dopamine while lowering norepinephrine.[24] Researchers have found that it changes brain waves as measured on EEG, promoting the relaxed and alert state associated with alpha waves.[25] That makes it unusual because it can sharpen mental focus and calm anxiety at the same time.

How to Use L-Theanine

In addition to rhodiola, described above, L-theanine is one of my most common treatments for anxiety and may help any of the seven types of anxiety. It is usually taken in doses from 50 to 200 mg once or twice daily. For severe anxiety, it may be taken three or four times per day. It is not habit-forming like so many antianxiety medications. There are no known drug interactions, but I recommend talking to your doctor before adding it to a medication. Side effects are minimal, but I have seen some patients experience mild sedation (if so, take at bedtime) or nausea (if so, take with food).

5-HTP

The best-studied of the "precursor strategies," wherein you try to increase production of a neurotransmitter by adding more of the raw materials, is 5-HTP. It is similar to tryptophan, which is the amino acid that gets converted into serotonin—5-HTP is the intermediate step in that process. Both are effective ways to boost serotonin levels, but tryptophan is more sedating so I usually reserve that for sleep problems. While 5-HTP can also help sleep, it may be used during the daytime as well because it is not usually sedating. Considerable research has shown that 5-HTP can reduce anxiety, both general and panic, as well as improve mood.[26]

How to Use 5-HTP

Whenever there are signs of serotonin deficiency (see above), adding 5-HTP may be helpful, especially if there are symptoms of depression along with anxiety. So many people are already taking SSRIs, however, that it complicates the use of 5-HTP. It is possible to get too much serotonin, a condition called *serotonin syndrome*, and that can be serious. *If you are already taking an SSRI, do not take 5-HTP without consulting your prescribing physician.*

I usually recommend a starting dose of 50 mg daily, increasing every few days as tolerated. Most people do well with 100–150 mg daily, but the dose may safely go as high as 300 mg per day if needed. It is usually best to take it divided into two or three doses throughout the day, but if it is sedating it may all be taken at night. However, a small number of people actually have trouble sleeping from 5-HTP, and should then take it early in the day.

It may be best absorbed if taken half an hour before meals, and that can also reduce carbohydrate cravings for people who have them. But if that is a hassle or causes stomach upset, it is fine to take it with meals.

NAC

NAC is short for n-acetylcysteine. You may have never heard of it before, but it has been used for years in emergency rooms for patients who are at risk for liver damage from something they have ingested (such as the common pain medication acetaminophen). It protects the liver for the same reason it protects the brain: it works as a powerful antioxidant, boosting levels of the body's own primary antioxidant—glutathione.

As researchers have realized the connection between glutamate/ GABA balance and anxiety conditions, they have begun experimenting with NAC. Recently it has been used with one of the most complex anxiety illnesses—the spectrum of compulsive disorders (including OCD). Remarkably, researchers have found that this simple and inexpensive nutritional supplement works for such hard-to-treat problems as pathological gambling and compulsive hair-pulling (trichotillomania).[27] Researchers at Yale are now conducting a placebo-controlled trial with patients whose OCD symptoms have not improved with other treatments.[28]

How to Use NAC

NAC typically comes in a dose of 600 mg and may be taken two or three times daily. Some of my patients have had mild headaches or stomach upset, but it is generally well tolerated, especially if you take it with food.

Taurine

Taurine is an amino acid that increases glycine and GABA to calm the brain, and it also protects the brain by reducing the harmful effects of excess glutamate.[29] You may be familiar with it, as it is added to some of the popular energy drinks such as Red Bull. Apparently the manufacturers see it as a means of further supporting someone during periods of extreme exertion, when taurine levels can become depleted. I don't recommend replenishing it through energy drinks, but you may calm your brain if you boost your taurine levels in safer ways.

How to Use Taurine

I consider taurine when someone has mood instability along with anxiety, but it may also be helpful for anxiety alone.

Taurine is usually taken in doses of 500 mg one to three times daily. It can cause slight drowsiness and if so may be taken at bedtime. It has also been known to reduce blood pressure, so you should use care if you are prone to hypotension or light-headedness. It may be taken with or without food.

Inositol

Inositol is often classified as a B vitamin, though technically it is not a vitamin since the body can produce it. Taken as a supplement, it has long been known to reduce general anxiety, panic, and OCD symptoms. Researchers found inositol to be just as effective as a popular antidepressant for panic disorder, and participants tolerated it well even at massive doses up to 18 grams per day.[30]

How to Use Inositol

Inositol is often recommended at a dose of about 1,500 mg daily, though in studies it has been used at much higher doses. Its side effects are mild, including occasional nausea or diarrhea, dizziness, fatigue, and headache. There has been a report of inositol worsening bipolar disorder, and I do not recommend it if you have that condition.

GABA

GABA has already been discussed as the neurotransmitter most responsible for calming down an overactive brain, and it is available as a nutritional supplement without prescription. Then why isn't it higher on my list of recommendations? If you take it by mouth most of it gets broken down before it gets to the brain, so it is not as useful as you might think. Still, a portion of it does appear to get into the brain, and some of GABA's calming effects may occur in the rest of the body, as with muscle relaxation. It has been shown in human studies to help create a relaxed alpha brain wave pattern even more effectively than L-theanine, and also to boost immune function in individuals who were subjected to stress.[31]

How to Use GABA

GABA may be taken in doses as small as 100 mg twice daily, up to 750 mg three times per day. If drowsiness occurs, take it just at bedtime. It may also occasionally cause headaches. You may find it more effective taken with a combination product containing some of the other nutrients discussed in this chapter.

DHEA

Dehydroepiandrosterone or DHEA is a steroid hormone produced in the adrenal glands, where cortisol and adrenaline are also made. It can be converted into testosterone and estrogen, and levels of DHEA are higher in men than in women. Because of its effects on the sex hormones, DHEA is not recommended for anyone with a gonadal tumor (prostate, ovarian, endometrial, breast, testicular) or at high risk for one (for example, with a family history of such tumors).

Despite these cautions, it remains available as a natural supplement without prescription, and it does appear to have strong effects against stress-related problems. More and more physicians are recommending it, particularly in midlife or beyond, when DHEA levels drop below normal. Supplementation has been shown to boost serotonin function, reduce cortisol, and improve mood by working through the GABA system.[32]

How to Use DHEA

I still recommend a cautious approach to DHEA, and suggest getting blood levels tested (which your doctor can order) before adding it as a supplement. If you are found to be low in DHEA, begin with a low dose of 5–10 mg daily and increase slowly under your doctor's supervision. Some clinicians recommend doses up to 50 mg or more. Levels can be monitored to be sure it doesn't get too high. And remember, do not use if you have ever had one of the above-mentioned tumors or if you are considered to be at high risk for developing one.

Therapeutic Herbs

There are many herbs that have been used safely for centuries to treat anxiety and stress-related problems. I will focus on the four that I consider to have the most research behind them: passionflower, valerian, St. John's wort, and ginkgo biloba. I use the first two most often for sleep, though they can have antianxiety effects as well when taken during the day.

There is one notable herb that I no longer include in my recommendations for anxiety: kava kava. It is perhaps the most effective and best-researched of all the herbs for anxiety. But in recent years there have been reports of liver failure associated with kava kava use, and it has been taken off the market in several herbal-friendly European countries. The FDA has not banned kava kava in the United States, but at this time I cannot recommend its use.

Each of the herbs described below may be used as a tincture or extract. Follow directions on the bottle, and remember to talk to your doctor before adding these, especially St. John's wort. As with all of the therapeutic supplements, I do not recommend them for long-term use. Many herbalists advise taking "herb holidays," particularly for the more potent herbs such as St. John's wort. To do so, you may use the herb for four to six months, and then take a couple of weeks or months off. Then resume it only if needed.

Passionflower

The name *passionflower* may give you the wrong impression of this calming herb, which I consider to be one of the best herbal remedies for anxiety and insomnia. Exactly how it works is unknown, but it may be a mild MAO inhibitor (thus increasing serotonin levels) or work through the GABA receptors.[33] It has been effective in treating anxiety without the dependence that can occur with many medications. One study compared passionflower with a drug called oxazepam, which is similar to Valium or Ativan. The herb was equally effective in treating anxiety with far less negative impact than the drug.[34]

The dosage varies by manufacturer. Look for a product containing at least 0.8 percent flavonoids and take as directed on the bottle. It may be used two or three times per day, and there are no known interactions with drugs or other serious risks. As with many herbal products, it may occasionally cause drowsiness, stomach upset, or mild headaches.

Valerian

Valerian has been called "natural Valium." It is not as effective as the prescription drugs, but it is also safer and non-addicting, and it may offer benefit for both anxiety and sleep. The plant contains some of the calming amino acids, such as arginine and GABA, and it is believed to work via GABA and serotonin receptors.[35] There was an older study combining valerian with St. John's wort and comparing that combination to the drug Valium for treatment of anxiety. The natural remedies actually came out on top.[36]

I usually recommend valerian for insomnia. If you would like to try it for anxiety, look for products that have been standardized to 0.8–1 percent valerenic acid. Doses vary widely by manufacturer, so take the amount suggested on the bottle. You may safely use it three or four times daily, and if it is going to help, its benefits should show up quickly, within a day or two. If it becomes too sedating (the most likely side effect), reduce the dose or take it all at bedtime.

St. John's wort

Although it is usually thought of as an antidepressant, St. John's wort can be quite effective for anxiety. It is believed to affect many of the primary neurotransmitters, including serotonin and dopamine, and also to decrease the stress hormones CRH and cortisol.[37] Small studies have found that St. John's wort works well for general anxiety and OCD, but more research is needed.[38]

St. John's wort is usually started at 300 mg three times daily, with doses going as high as 1,800 mg per day. Look for a product standardized to 0.3 percent hypericins. Do not add St. John's wort to another antidepressant, and avoid it if taking birth control pills or while pregnant.

It can interact with some medications, such as digoxin or Coumadin, so be sure to talk with your doctor first before adding to any medication.

It may take six to eight weeks for St. John's wort to work, so be patient. And be careful with the sun—it may make you more sensitive to it.

Ginkgo Biloba

You may think of ginkgo as a memory enhancer, and that is where it has been studied the most. But one reason why it may improve memory is because it can help normalize the stress response and thereby protect against the memory loss that can occur from prolonged exposure to cortisol.[39] There has been some research using ginkgo for anxiety, with positive results.[40]

I don't usually recommend ginkgo as a first-line treatment for anxiety, but if you are going through a period of intense stress, or if your memory and concentration seem to be affected by anxiety, it may be a great support. It is considered quite safe with very few side effects, which may include mild headaches, gastric upset, or dizziness. It may increase risk of bleeding if you are taking Coumadin.

The usual dose is 60 mg twice a day, and it should be standardized to 24 percent flavone glycosides (or ginkgolides). It may take six to eight weeks or more to see noticeable results.

Putting Together a Resilient Supplement Plan

After reading about all of these supplements, you may imagine yourself taking a fistful of pills each day and spending a small fortune doing so. Supplements can be expensive, and that is one of their limitations. I try to be very sensitive to costs, as well as to the quantity of supplements that I prescribe. When I see patients, we can often streamline their supplements, taking out things that are redundant or less important. As I said earlier in the chapter, I view these as supplements that can support your physiology during hard times, rather than as the answer to the problems of stress.

Let me describe how I put together a supplement plan, referring back to Jessica, whom I introduced in chapter 2, as an example. I begin with the first three foundational supplements, which I recommend to everyone in the Resilience Training Program: a multivitamin (or B complex), vitamin D_3, and omega-3s. Jessica was relatively young and healthy and spent plenty of time outdoors, so I didn't get a vitamin D level for her. I would recommend the blood test in people of color or those of advancing age, or if there are several illnesses, chronic pain, or other symptoms that are not responsive to treatment.

Next, I consider the other two foundational supplements, which I usually add for anxiety problems: the minerals and the tonic herb rhodiola. Whenever there is anxiety coupled with insomnia, physical restlessness, or muscle tension, I recommend magnesium. Since Jessica is a woman, I gave her a supplement containing both calcium and magnesium. She got plenty of zinc in her multivitamin, so we didn't add more, but if she had failed to improve, I might have later checked her zinc levels. And since she had such a range of symptoms for so long, I encouraged her to add rhodiola. I view that as a long-term support for an overly strained stress system, which may be unnecessary for temporary or short-term stresses.

After starting these basic supplements, I often wait a couple of weeks before adding more things, especially if someone is just beginning to make dietary changes and add exercise and meditation to their program. But in Jessica's case, her symptoms were too severe to wait, and she was already on the SSRI medication Zoloft and having problems with it. I don't always recommend coming off medication, but it clearly was not helping her and I agreed with her assessment that it was making some of her symptoms worse. So we began reducing her medication, cutting the dose by 25 percent every two weeks and watching to be sure that she had no withdrawal symptoms.

At the same time, she needed some immediate relief. Whenever that is the case, I prefer to start with just one or two of the therapeutic supplements, usually choosing one amino acid (L-theanine, 5-HTP, taurine, or GABA) and perhaps one therapeutic herb. If the main type of anxiety is panic, I may recommend inositol. Or if compulsive symptoms are predominant, I would likely choose NAC.

Jessica had developed such a range of symptoms (she had most of the seven types of anxiety by the time I saw her) that she needed a broad spectrum of support. So I recommended a combination product that contained NAC, green tea extract, and taurine. And since we were reducing her Zoloft and I felt she had signs of serotonin deficiency, I added 50 mg of 5-HTP (but only when her Zoloft dose had been decreased by 50 percent).

Jessica's story is a happy one. She felt immediate relief, which may have been due to her feeling hopeful again, coupled with reducing her medication. When I saw her again in two weeks, she felt 80 percent better, and things kept improving over the next few weeks. Now she feels better than she has in years, calmer even than before the car accident. I am sure that balancing her brain chemistry was responsible for much of her improvement.

Jessica was able to get off her medication, and she felt so much better that she considered leaving it at that. But she was also committed to preventing this from happening again, so she went through the entire Resilience Training Program. She learned how her thoughts and emotions worked and how she could keep herself calm by becoming more skilled with them, how to eat to keep her brain and body chemistry balanced, and what to do to sustain her energy throughout her life, which remained stressful. In the next chapter we will look more closely at how you, too, can manage your energy.

6

Step 2: Manage Your Energy

Why Recharging Your Body Is Key to Sustaining a Healthy Mind

The energy of the mind is the essence of life.

—ARISTOTLE

Key Points

- Mental energy, like physical energy, can become depleted by the chronic stress response. To restore it, we must first address some consequences of long-term stress that can impair energy production.
- There are a few key nutrients that often become deficient with age, illness, or chronic stress. Replenishing them may quickly restore energy *and* the ability to make more of it.
- The economics of energy are like good investing: spend it wisely and you will get even more of it. Your best investment is regular exercise, which not only protects the cells but also makes them better energy producers.

SCOTT IS a psychotherapist who heard me speak at a workshop and felt inspired by the idea that resilience can be regained no matter how long symptoms have been present or how chronic the stress response has become. He himself has struggled with anxiety since his late teenage years, and he has been depressed on and off his entire life. Now in his early fifties, he has developed several additional problems: he is overweight, has preclinical diabetes that he has tried unsuccessfully to manage with diet, and has already had one mild heart attack. He came to see me after the end of a stressful twenty-five-year marriage that was especially rocky as they approached their separation and divorce.

Now financially strapped and responsible for their three adolescent children, his stress level had never been higher, nor his reserves lower. He had already been through years of treatment with psychotherapy and medication, with limited benefit, and he wasn't looking for more of the same. What he wanted now, more than anything, was fairly simple: he wanted reason to hope.

Scott had undergone decades of unhealthy stress and had developed many of the consequences that can occur if the stress response is not shut down. As you will see in Scott's story, chronic stress feeds upon itself. It creates its own set of physiological problems that, in turn, add even more stress to the body.

Despite being an athlete in his youth, Scott was not a fan of exercise and his weight had increased over the years to the point that he was now considered to be obese. Most of the weight had gone to his belly, a pattern commonly seen with men, but increasingly with women as well. Moreover, his doctor had recently told him that he had preclinical diabetes—his blood sugar had risen and his own insulin was no longer effectively dealing with it, so that he was now faced with adding a new medication to treat this. And his real wake-up call occurred when he suffered a mild heart attack and his doctor told him he had to work on lowering both his weight and his stress level. The heart attack, combined with his other symptoms, suggested that his body was not only stressed but inflamed as well.

Scott's story is incredibly common. He was caught in a complex cycle that he could not seem to undo: after living for years under perpetual stress, his body had changed in ways that created even more harmful stress reactions—and these changes kept the stress reaction going.

Scott had developed a common triumvirate of stress-related issues:

- **Oxidative stress.** This is stress at the cellular level. You don't see it, but the consequences include damage to the parts of the cells that produce energy—the very energy that could help stop the stress spiral.
- **Blood sugar dysregulation.** Loading up on sugar or refined carbohydrates strains both the hormones involved and the cells' capacity to process sugar. This further erodes the ability to produce energy, and signals the adrenals to keep the stress hormones coming.
- **Body-wide inflammation.** Caused by the two problems listed above, among other factors, inflammation creates harmful chemicals that continue to damage important tissues, perpetuating a number of diseases, including heart disease, depression, and anxiety.

These interrelated problems make it harder to recover from anxiety or stress, or from any chronic illness, for that matter. One reason that they are so insidious is that they rob you of energy, mental focus, and motivation—the very tools that are required to improve your health. So until these problems are addressed, the cycle goes on and on.

They can be quite complex, and may require medical treatment if they have become entrenched, as they had for Scott. But to a large degree, they *can* be reversed. It is best to deal with them as soon as possible, but as Scott found out, it is never too late to begin.

The Energy Thieves

Oxidative Stress: Rusting from the Inside Out

Energy is a renewable resource, within our bodies as well as in the larger ecosystem. We are not aware of it, but there are millions of tiny factories inside of us that are constantly producing the energy that we need to keep ourselves going every day that we are alive. Known as *mitochondria*, they are found inside every cell in varying numbers, depending upon how much energy that particular cell needs.

Which part of the body do you think has the highest concentration of mitochondria? It is the brain, which uses a full 20 percent of the body's main fuel—glucose (blood sugar). The rest of the body can use other sources of energy, like protein or fat. But the brain relies upon glucose as its power source. If that energy supply begins running low—if we become hypoglycemic (have low blood sugar)—then the brain sends out ever-louder alarms to the rest of the body to get it some fuel. We experience that as anxiety.

Glucose gets turned into useable energy through a complex metabolic process called the Krebs cycle. This requires oxygen, which is where we get the terms *oxidation* and *oxidative stress*. The end result of this cycle is a molecule called adenosine triphosphate (ATP), which is packed full of energy for the brain cells to use to produce neurotransmitters, copy segments of DNA, or whatever else is needed for that cell to carry out its functions. At the same time, there are waste products that come out of this process, including carbon dioxide and water, which are easily eliminated.

But other by-products of metabolism, known as *free radicals*, can be harmful if not neutralized. We see this happen in the outside world, as when cut fruit becomes brown or copper turns green. Oxidation can even cause the breakdown of hard metals, which we call rust.

Inside our bodies, too, free radicals are powerful and can be destructive. They are very unstable molecules because they are missing an electron. In order to stabilize themselves, they attack the nearest available molecule and steal one of *its* electrons, harming that other molecule in the process.

The mitochondria themselves are very vulnerable to being damaged by free radicals if not protected. If enough damage occurs, the cell itself may die. When a great number of cells are destroyed, you can imagine how any number of diseases can result.

Our bodies have their own means of dealing with this—the antioxidants. They're like the workers who go in to clean up unstable waste material in a nuclear power plant. But sometimes our own defenses become overwhelmed—either because there are too many free radicals or because we have too few antioxidants to protect against them. The latter is best addressed through diet (eating colorful fruits and vegetables). We will also discuss a few powerful antioxidant supplements later in this chapter.

What causes an increase in free radicals, and how can we reduce them to protect the mitochondria as well as the nerve cells themselves?

Exposure to toxins of any kind may increase free radicals within the body. Those include environmental pollutants, cigarette smoke, heavy metals such as mercury, herbicides and pesticides, and even some household cleaners. Of course, we can't completely avoid toxins, but we should do so as much as possible, and eat many of the protective foods described in chapter 4. This is also one of the best reasons to eat organic foods, because they are raised without harmful chemicals.

Free radicals are also made in the normal process of metabolism. If we eat too many calories, or if we are under stress for long periods of time, then we will make more of these harmful by-products. It may be wise under those circumstances to add additional antioxidant protection, but it's even wiser to deal with the root causes. Two of the most common triggers of free radical damage are insulin resistance and inflammation.

Insulin Resistance: Overloaded with Sugar

Carbohydrates are broken down within the intestines to glucose, which then travels throughout the body in our blood. Before it can be converted into energy, though, glucose has to be taken inside the cells where the mitochondria reside. Insulin is the hormone that makes that happen, by giving a message to the cell to let the sugar in. If you put too much strain on the insulin system, the cells become resistant to its message. Then the pancreas produces more insulin in order to coax the cells to take in more blood sugar. Over time, the cells become less and less responsive to insulin's effects.

That's what happened to Scott. He had always had a sweet tooth, but as he aged and became less active, he burned fewer calories. He gained weight but didn't change his eating habits. Though he wasn't aware of it, his blood sugar levels began to soar after he overate, and that forced his pancreas to work extra hard, making more insulin to try to get the sugar out of the bloodstream and into the cells. After years of getting urgent messages to bring in more sugar, his cells began to weary of insulin and ignored its call. That left even *more* sugar in his bloodstream, raising a signal for yet more insulin. With time, no matter how much insulin there was, the cells became deaf to its message, and Scott had become dangerously close to having full-fledged diabetes.

Meanwhile, Scott felt more and more fatigued and unable to focus.

Because of his ongoing stress, he had become really inefficient at producing energy. He had plenty of fuel, but couldn't get it into the cells or the mitochondria where it could be used.

What Does Stress Have to Do with It?

Cortisol levels rise with any stressful event, even normal ones. This rise is *supposed* to increase hunger, because the fight-or-flight reaction can use up energy reserves and they need to be restored. Cortisol also counteracts insulin's signal to take sugar out of the bloodstream.[1] When the body goes into fight-or-flight mode, it may need more fuel at any time. Having sugar in the bloodstream makes for easy access.

But with prolonged stress, Scott's cortisol remained high, continually increasing both his hunger and blood sugar. The foods he craved were sweets and refined carbs—the "comfort foods." Though he had a lot of glucose in his bloodstream, it wouldn't go into the cells, so the brain kept sending distress calls to get more sugar.

That's one of the reasons Scott kept eating too much. He criticized himself for this: "Look at me, I'm overweight and I can't stop bingeing—I just don't have any discipline." It wasn't that he was undisciplined. Scott was simply responding to the compelling order his body gave him to keep eating refined carbs.

Most of his weight gain was around his midsection, a sign that he had become insulin resistant.[2] He didn't know it, but the more weight he added around his belly, the harder it became to lose weight—or to feel good. That is because visceral adipose tissue, as belly fat is known, actually produces hormones—it's like adding a new endocrine gland to your body. As you can imagine, these are not healthy, helpful hormones. Visceral fat produces hormones that add to stress, appetite, and inflammation. What's more, it worsens insulin resistance, making it even harder to lose weight or to feel good.[3]

Being unable to effectively process glucose, Scott couldn't make the energy he needed, and so he felt constantly tired, run-down, and unable to focus. He was caught in a common negative spiral: stress elevates cortisol; cortisol increases hunger and alters insulin and blood sugar, causing weight gain around the middle; belly fat itself secretes stress hormones, causing even more weight gain; the resulting insulin resistance adds yet more stress, creating more free radicals, keeping cortisol levels high . . . and so the vicious cycle goes.[4]

This pattern can result in a condition known as *metabolic syndrome*, placing one at high risk for heart disease and type 2 diabetes, as happened to Scott. He is not alone: according to the National Institutes of Health, nearly 50 million Americans have metabolic syndrome.[5] That should give health planners great incentive for putting vastly more resources into prevention programs. Allowing this problem to grow unchecked will create a great deal of suffering—and treating the long-term health consequences will be unimaginably expensive.

Obesity and heart disease are not the only problems that result from blood sugar dysregulation. There is growing recognition that insulin resistance and metabolic syndrome affect the brain as well, and are now thought to be one of the key risk factors for depression and other mental health problems.[6]

What Is Metabolic Syndrome?

The American Heart Association and the National Heart, Lung and Blood Institute define metabolic syndrome as meeting 3 or more of the following criteria:

- Abdominal obesity: waist circumference is greater than 40 inches in men and greater than 35 inches in women. (A more sensitive measure is the waist-to-hip ratio. Using a measuring tape, measure around the belly just above the navel. Take a second measurement at the widest part of your hips. Calculate the ratio (waist divided by hip). In men, this ratio should be less than 0.9, and in women less than 0.8.)

- Elevated triglycerides: 150 mg/dL or higher.
- Reduced HDL cholesterol: less than 40 mg/dL for men, and less than 50 mg/dL for women.
- High blood pressure: 130/85 mm Hg or higher.
- Increased fasting blood glucose: 100 mg/dL or higher.

Source: American Heart Association (www.americanheart.org)

Chronic Inflammation: Fire in the Belly (and the Heart, and the Brain)

One of the primary ways that blood sugar dysregulation impacts mental health is to promote inflammation in the brain as well as throughout the body. Inflammation, like stress, is a normal physical reaction—healthy up to a point. It is intended to protect against injury, infection, or invasion by something foreign to your body. But if the reaction is too strong or goes on too long, it can become damaging. When inflammation is prolonged, it may compound the initial problem by turning up the stress response even further, creating even higher levels of cortisol with all of its consequences.

In recent years, systemic inflammation (meaning inflammation that occurs throughout the body) has been linked to most chronic diseases, including Alzheimer's, diabetes, heart disease, cancer, and depression.[7] Inflammation does its damage through chemicals called *cytokines*, which can quickly lead to a loss of energy and more gradually to a negative mood. Cytokines also create anxiety and memory loss, perhaps through toxicity to the neurons and by disrupting neuroplasticity.[8]

Systemic inflammation is insidious because we often don't recognize that it is there. We can see it if it is on or near the skin, because it creates redness, heat, and swelling, not to mention pain. When inflammation is inside the body it is equally destructive but hidden to us. There are good ways to tone it down once it's discovered, so the key is often to simply recognize its presence. In addition to the signs below, many doctors rely upon a simple blood test that measures C-reactive protein, or CRP. This protein is produced by the liver in reaction to systemic inflammation and tells you that inflammation is present. If you have some of the signs listed below, consider getting a high-sensitivity CRP blood test through your doctor's office.

Signs of Inflammation

If you have two or more of the following, you may have body-wide inflammation:

- Allergies, sinusitis
- Asthma, bronchitis
- Arthritis, joint pain, or injuries that are slow to heal (e.g., tendinitis)
- Gum disease (gingivitis)
- Skin problems, including acne, eczema, and psoriasis
- Migraines or cluster headaches
- Bowel disease (irritable bowel, colitis, inflammatory bowel disease)
- Heart disease

- Diabetes or central obesity (elevated waist-to-hip ratio; see above)
- Depression

Renewing Energy

If you are energy deficient, focus first on these four areas before moving on to the rest of the Resilience Training Program:

1. Follow the Resilient Diet (chapter 4)
2. Consider one or more key supplements (see below)
3. Begin a gentle exercise program (see below)
4. Tone down the stress response (beginning with chapter 7)

If you show signs of metabolic syndrome or systemic inflammation, you should start by consulting your doctor, because the consequences of ignoring these conditions can be high. Whether you require medical treatment or not, it is crucial to begin with these lifestyle changes now. They may be able to reverse, or at least slow the progression of these conditions.

The Resilient Diet is a great place to start, because it addresses all of these problems simultaneously. If you need some motivation to help you get started, consider a recent article in the *Journal of the American College of Cardiology*.[9] The authors' review of the dietary literature led them to conclude that a single meal high in saturated fats and refined carbohydrates can cause oxidative stress, hyperglycemia, and inflammation—*a single meal!* Likewise, choosing healthier foods such as those in the Resilient Diet can have an *immediate* positive effect on your health. So every single time you eat, you have a fresh chance to create a more resilient brain.

Here are some of the dietary suggestions to emphasize if you need to confront the energy thieves.

For Oxidative Stress

- Eat fewer overall calories.
- Pay special attention to fruits and vegetables:
- Eat cruciferous vegetables every day (broccoli, kale, collard greens, cauliflower, Brussels sprouts, cabbage, bok choy, broccoli rabe, broccolini). They help protect against toxins.
- Try to have two colorful fruits and vegetables (green, yellow, red, orange, blue, and purple) at each meal, or at least every day. Pomegranates, red wine, tea, and dark chocolate also contain potent antioxidants, which protect against free radical damage.

For Insulin Resistance

- Eat fewer calories overall, but eat small amounts regularly (every three to six hours).
- Include high-quality protein (e.g., lean meats, low-fat cheese, egg whites, fish, whey protein, or other protein powders) with each meal and snack (including breakfast). This helps keep blood sugar stable.
- Pay special attention to carbs—they are the primary cause of insulin resistance.
- Reduce the amount of calories that come from carbohydrates.
- Switch gradually from simple carbs (sugar, white breads, pastas, pastries, most snack foods) to complex carbs (fruits,

grains, beans, and root vegetables that still have lots of fiber).

- Choose carbs that have a lower glycemic index—that means that they get converted into sugar more slowly.
- Get rid of high fructose corn syrup—but *don't* replace it with artificial sweeteners!
- Use cinnamon (¼–½ teaspoon daily as a spice, or taken as an extract), which may enhance insulin function and reduce blood sugar.[10]
- Vinegar (1–2 tablespoons) with a meal will slow the spike in blood sugar because acetic acid slows the rate at which the stomach empties.[11] Mix it with olive oil for a healthy salad dressing.

For Inflammation

- Reduce intake of pro-inflammatory foods, which can aggravate inflammation, especially refined carbohydrates and red meats and other animal products.
- Pay special attention to fats. Improving the ratio of healthy to unhealthy fat is the best means to shut off the cascade of inflammatory cytokines.
- Cut back on saturated fats found in red meats and dairy (butter, cheese, ice cream, whole-milk products).
- Favor grass-fed over corn-fed animal products.
- Use olive or walnut oils.
- Eat plenty of cold-water fish, nuts, and seeds.
- Add anti-inflammatory spices such as ginger and turmeric.[12]
- Look for food sensitivities, a common hidden cause of inflammation. You can try an elimination diet or get a blood

test. You may wish to see a qualified health practitioner to guide you.

Energy Boosters

If you need extra help getting going, consider these energy-boosting supplements.

PURPOSE	SUPPLEMENT	TYPICAL DOSAGE	COMMENTS
Cellular energy production	Alpha-lipoic acid (ALA)	300–600 mg daily.	Levels decrease with age. A potent antioxidant; also helps energy production and improves glucose metabolism.[13]
	Acetyl L-carnitine	500–1,000 mg daily.	Aids mitochondrial production of ATP. Also has antioxidant effects.[14]
	Coenzyme Q_{10} (coQ_{10})	30–200 mg daily.	Works within mitochondria to help energy production; synergistic with ALA.[15]

	D-ribose	3–5 grams up to 3 times daily.	A sugar that is easily converted into ATP. Can improve muscle function and exercise tolerance and reduce oxidative stress.[16]
Additional antioxidant protection	Green tea extract or EGCG	300–500 mg extract twice daily, or 150–350 mg EGCG twice a day.	A strong antioxidant may promote cell health and blood sugar regulation and also reduce inflammation.[17]
	Grapeseed or red wine extracts	100–200 mg daily, with procyanidolic value of 95.	Contains proanthocyanidins, especially good at neutralizing free radicals; these may give red wine (and resveratrol) its purported health benefits.[18]
	Pycnogenol	50–100 mg twice daily.	Reported benefits in all three areas: antioxidant, blood sugar regulation, and inflammation.[19]

Glucose/insulin balancing	Glucomannan fiber	2–3 grams taken with water before meals.	An unusually viscous dietary fiber, it reduces glucose and insulin surges after meals.[20]
	Chromium picolinate	200 mcg up to three times daily.	Improves insulin function, reduces carbohydrate cravings.[21]
Anti-inflammatory	Omega-3/fish oil	1,000–4,000 mg daily.	Reduces inflammation by improving prostaglandin function. Also helps with insulin resistance.[22]
	Turmeric extract (curcumin)	300–600 mg two or three times daily; look for 95 percent curcuminoids.	Antioxidant, anti-inflammatory. Protects brain from stress and injury.[23]

The above supplements are arranged by their function, rather than their order of preference. However, I would recommend beginning with the first three supplements listed (alpha-lipoic acid, acetyl L-carnitine, and coenzyme Q_{10}), because they work synergistically and together may address many of the causes for energy depletion. You may wish to try those for a few weeks before adding more supplements.

They can be especially helpful in middle age and beyond, as these natural body chemicals tend to decrease with age.

If you have a great deal of muscle fatigue or just cannot seem to exercise because of tiredness, consider adding D-ribose just before physical activity. Or divide the dose, taking half before and half after exercising. It works quickly, so you should know within a few days if it is going to help you enough to warrant the price, which can be fairly steep. It may be worth it if it helps you get started with an exercise program, and after a few weeks of regular exercise you may no longer need it.

The antioxidants help protect against free radical damage—but remember, the best source of antioxidants comes from a diet rich in brightly colored plant foods. Also, if you are taking a quality multivitamin, you should be getting fairly good antioxidant protection. Any of the three antioxidants listed (green tea extract, grapeseed extract, or Pycnogenol) can be added, at least temporarily, to offer additional protection during times of stress or illness. Because of cost, I would recommend trying them one at a time or getting them in a combined supplement. Give each of them at least four to six weeks as a trial to determine if it is helpful to you.

The next two supplements are intended only for those who have blood sugar problems, particularly if there is insulin resistance or metabolic syndrome. Glucomannan is a fiber and chromium is a mineral, and both are meant to help stabilize blood sugar. If you have these conditions, you should also be working with your health care provider.

The anti-inflammatory supplements (omega-3s and turmeric or curcumin) may also improve blood sugar metabolism. Omega-3s are among the foundational supplements recommended in chapter 5, but I list them again because they have such strong anti-inflammatory effects and should definitely be part of the regimen when inflammation is present. Turmeric is a spice that offers potent brain protection and can be taken in a concentrated form often called curcumin.

Resilient Movement: Restoring Power from Within

Imagine a drug that was inexpensive, had no negative side effects when used properly, helped everyone who used it, prevented most chronic illness, slowed the aging process, improved sleep, reduced stress, protected the brain, lifted mood, boosted self-esteem, and even enhanced one's sex life—it would be more popular than Prozac!

As Sue Masemer, my colleague in the Resilience Training Program, likes to say, "Exercise is medicine." Sue is a top-notch exercise physiologist, and she evaluated Scott, as she does every participant in our program. Sue also works with professional athletes, so she understands the full range of interest in and experience with exercise.

For many people, the term *exercise* has an unpleasant ring to it. They think of exercise as arduous, recall the many times they've tried and failed to keep a program going, or compare themselves to others at a health club who look more fit than they could ever dream of being.

Scott was among that group. He knew that he *should* exercise, but he had become so sluggish and carried so many negative messages about it that he just could not get started. Sue shared with Scott the most important thing to know about exercise: *what really matters is that you do something—almost anything—that moves your body.*

One of Scott's obstacles was the belief that it would take months of pain before he could hope to start feeling better. But just as you can improve your blood chemistry with a single meal, you can also boost energy, mental focus, and mood with a single simple workout. That was the conclusion of a study done with people being treated for depression. A single thirty-minute session of moderate activity (walking on a treadmill) gave participants a quick mental and emotional lift.[24] It's hard to be in a bad mood while exercising.

Those results are not surprising. Evidence keeps showing that exercise can be as effective as antidepressants in treating major depression, and adding exercise can even help those who fail to respond to antidepressant medications.[25] As you might expect, it also helps ease anxiety. Aerobic exercise can even reduce the sensitivity to certain physical sensations that may lead to panic attacks, such as increased breathing and heart rates.[26] Apparently, creating some of the sensations through exercise trains the brain to see them as normal, rather than as reason to set off the alarms.

Still, Scott was not convinced. "I'm middle-aged and overweight and have already had a heart attack. Maybe if I'd started ten or twenty years ago, it would have done me more good." But recent research should encourage even the most resigned couch potatoes—*it is not too late to start*.

In fact, midlife may be the key period for reaping the long-term benefits from exercise, even if it wasn't a regular part of your life before. In a study done in Scandinavia, it was shown that exercise in middle-aged men can reverse metabolic syndrome, especially if combined with changes in diet.[27] And a 2009 study in the *British Medical Journal* found that sedentary men who increased their activity at age fifty lengthened their life spans—to the same level as those who had always exercised.[28]

Why does exercise have such powerful effects on stress-related problems? Like diet, it may have to do with gene expression. Researchers from Yale discovered an exercise-related gene located in the hippocampus, right in the middle of the brain's fear circuitry. This gene regulates a key growth factor known as VGF, which acts as a powerful antidepressant, perhaps by influencing nerve growth and plasticity.[29]

Exercise does it all when it comes to dealing with stress-related conditions. It protects cells from oxidation, helps normalize blood sugar, reverses metabolic syndrome, decreases inflammation, treats depression, and promotes new brain cell survival, growth, and learning.[30] It even increases insulin receptors, helps normalize cortisol levels, and boosts BDNF, the brain's growth factor.[31] Exercise *is* a wonder drug.

Even Scott was coming around, realizing that he needed to address his long aversion to exercise and beginning to believe that he could do so. His next question was: "How much do I have to do?"

Before addressing that central question, let's consider the evolution of fear and the fight-or-flight reaction. Remember that we are well designed to experience fear, that it is normal and even healthy when it is short-lived. For the sake of survival, it has always been necessary to generate short, intense bursts of activity, as would be required to run away or to stay and fight. Those brief periods of vigorous movement not only were necessary for survival but also helped keep the energy system at peak efficiency and return the stress hormones back to normal.

Movement was mostly about survival. Even when there weren't immediate threats, there was the need to gather food and provide shelter. There wasn't "exercise" as we have come to know it. There was just activity built into the normal course of the day—a lot of activity. No one was an athlete—or perhaps *everyone* was an athlete. People were moving nearly all the time, hunting, gathering, or just roaming.

As societies evolved to more stable, less nomadic lives, most people became farmers. Even in this country, until the last fifty or a hundred years, nearly everyone was involved with agriculture or in some way made a living by using their bodies. Very few people sat at a desk all day. The idea of carving out thirty minutes a few times a week to "exercise" is really a new phenomenon. It is born out of necessity because 90 percent of us now sit at a desk all day long, then drive home (sitting again), eat a quickly prepared meal, and sit some more in front of the TV or computer. "Exercise" as we have come to know it isn't really natural. It is something we have to do because we have given up most natural forms of movement.

So I invite you to think of three different kinds of movement:

1. **Exercise.** Intentional exertion done to maintain physical fitness—such as jogging, using elliptical trainers, or lifting weights.
2. **Non-exercise.** Any routine type of movement built into the day, including walking, biking to work, taking the stairs, house or yard work, or even pacing or fidgeting.
3. **Mindful movement.** An activity that requires greater awareness of the body, such as yoga or t'ai chi, or that involves learning skilled movements, such as dancing or playing a musical instrument.

Each of these is important, and each has a slightly different benefit. Ideally, you would do some of each, but the main point is to do more of *any* of them. The one thing you shouldn't do is to remain sedentary.

Exercise

Back to Scott's question: "How much do I need to do?" The U.S. Department of Health and Human Services recently convened a panel of experts and came up with new recommendations, the 2008 Physical Activity Guidelines for Americans. Most fitness experts have endorsed these guidelines, and I think they are very sound as well.

Weekly Minimum Exercise Guidelines for Adults

- At least 2½ hours of moderate-intensity aerobic activity per week
- *Or* 75 minutes of vigorous-intensity aerobic activity per week
- *Plus* muscle-strengthening activity at least two days per week

Source: http://www.cdc.gov/physicalactivity/everyone/guidelines/adults.html

Remember, these are *exercise* guidelines, so the intent is to push your heart rate beyond its resting rate by doing an aerobic activity. "Moderate intensity" is defined as breaking a sweat and being able to talk but not sing. A brisk walk, easy biking, playing doubles tennis, or mowing the lawn should suffice. "Vigorous intensity" involves getting the heart rate to a higher level and breathing hard enough so that you can only say a few words at a time. This may require jogging, using an elliptical trainer, or playing a sport such as singles tennis or racquetball. Whatever you do should be sustained for at least ten minutes at a time. Of course you can do more than two and a half hours per week. That is considered a minimum, and more is better—at least up to a point.

Muscle strengthening is an important part of these guidelines. Strength training can greatly reduce joint problems and injury as we age, and helps right away with reducing stress and boosting self-esteem. The guidelines suggest working with every major muscle group: legs, hips, back, chest, abdomen, shoulders, and arms. There are a lot of options: using free weights or weight machines, resistance bands, or your own body weight (as in push-ups, sit-ups, and pull-ups). To get the most out of it, they suggest using enough resistance that it is hard to do more than eight to twelve repetitions without assistance. Note that yoga and heavy gardening also count as resistance activities.

Be sure to be guided by your physician regarding how to start and how quickly to increase your activity levels, especially if you have any of the following:

- A known heart condition
- Chest discomfort with or without physical exertion
- Loss of balance due to dizziness
- Loss of consciousness
- Joint problems
- Medication for high blood pressure or heart problems
- Any other reason you should not do physical activity

Source: Physical Activity Readiness Questionnaire, developed by the British Columbia Ministry of Health

Non-Exercise

If you follow the above guidelines, you will exercise two to three hours per week. That leaves roughly 165 hours per week (more than 98 percent of the time) when you *won't* be exercising. You can see the problem. We evolved to be moving most of the day—not exercising, but moving. Instead, we sit.

Researchers at the Mayo Clinic use the term *NEAT* (non-exercise activity thermogenesis) to refer to extra movement that is not done for fitness purposes. As you might guess, there is a huge spectrum in the amount of non-exercise movement done by different people. In fact, one of the biggest differences between those who are obese and those who are not is in how much each group moves during the day. Movement burns calories, even if it is taking a stroll, tapping your toes, or moving your hands as you talk. Even chewing gum burns a few calories.[32]

The best way for most people to add more movement is to walk.

It doesn't have to be a fitness walk, though that is good, too. It just means being on your feet often, getting up from the chair for an errand, taking a leisurely stroll in a park, or even pacing about while waiting for someone. Walking is cheap, it is easy, and most people can get started without risking injury.

I suggest getting up from your desk or chair several times per day to take a ten-minute stroll. It's even better if you walk fast enough to raise your heart rate, and if you sustain that for thirty minutes or more. But the main thing is to move, and to move often. It may help to set up a system, such as an alarm on your cell phone or electronic planner, to remind you to get up and move every hour and a half to two hours.

Mindful Movement

Any movement that you do, you can do with greater awareness. You can incorporate mindfulness into your ten-minute strolls, thirty-minute bike rides, or twice-weekly weight training. But some activities demand greater awareness, and the resulting mind-body integration offers more benefits for the brain than do other forms of movement.

If you are struggling with anxiety or going through a stressful time, I strongly encourage you to find a yoga class. If you have never done yoga, it should be easy to find a beginning class that you can do. The combination of slow movement, gentle stretching, and relaxed breathing is just what your body craves to help it calm down.

T'ai chi is another good option for calming stress. Like yoga, its movements are gentle and slow, and it usually incorporates mindful breathing. There is often an emphasis on flowing movement and balance. Also, it requires you to learn a number of new positions, almost like learning a complex dance. That new learning helps create more brain growth and may improve mental focus and calm overactive parts of the brain. Qigong is even simpler to learn and focuses more on breathing and on the meditative aspect of the movements, making it ideal for stress and anxiety.

Remember that overall brain health requires new learning and growth. Yoga and t'ai chi offer that, but so does any physical activity that involves complex movements. Think of an activity that you might really enjoy, such as golfing, dancing, picking up a musical instrument, balancing on one foot, juggling—anything that sounds fun and challenges you at the same time. Count it as exercise if you'd like—just find ways of moving that appeal to you so that you will keep doing them.

Scott found himself drawn most naturally to the non-exercise form of movement. He began very slowly, taking a five-minute walk just a couple of times per day. Since it didn't feel like work to him, he stayed with it, gradually adding more minutes and walking more frequently. Before long, he started feeling energetic enough to add an easy bike ride twice a week, and at the suggestion of our training staff, he started using a balance ball to do some simple resistance training.

Now one year later, Scott has dropped twenty-five pounds and his blood sugars are stable without medication. He takes the foundational supplements (a multivitamin, omega-3s, and vitamin D_3) along with rhodiola and L-theanine. In addition, he takes a supplement combining alpha-lipoic acid, acetyl L-carnitine, and coQ_{10}, which he thinks has really helped his energy.

Balancing brain chemistry and managing energy can go a long way toward getting you back on track, as was the case for Scott. The long-term solution still requires that you normalize the stress response.

As a side benefit to all that he was doing, Scott says that he is sleeping better than he has in years—a clear sign that his stress hormone levels are down. In the next chapter we will look more specifically at measures you can take to tone the sympathetic nervous system and calm both body and mind.

7

Step 3: Align with Nature

How to Tame Your Mind and Ease Your Anxiety

Tension is who you think you should be. Relaxation is who you are.

—CHINESE PROVERB

Key Points

- Nature is built upon rhythms and cycles: day followed by night, activity followed by rest, tension followed by relaxation.
- It is completely natural, and within your reach, to recover from stress every day.
- Sometimes doing nothing is the most restorative action you can take.
- Quality sleep is a powerfully protective cornerstone of resilience.

PICTURE A quiet afternoon on the African savannah, a herd of impala grazing serenely, looking as though they hadn't a care in the world. Suddenly their peacefulness is shattered as a cheetah races into their midst, scattering the impala like dust. The cheetah locks its sights on one young impala, whose desperate maneuvers are no match for the oncoming cheetah. All too quickly, it is over. The impala lies defeated on the ground with the cheetah's jaws clamped around its neck.

Then, surprisingly, the cheetah releases its grip and slowly walks away. Apparently it is not hungry and seems to have lost interest, leaving for dead the body of the fallen impala. In a few moments, the impala begins to move and then miraculously stands and shakes its body for a minute or so, as if it were shaking off the fear. You watch, amazed, as it wanders off to rejoin its group, looking as though nothing much had happened.

This describes a video shown by psychologist Peter Levine, who does research on trauma and anxiety. He describes what happened to the impala as a normal, automatic reaction to an overwhelming threat. Known as the *freezing response*, it is a last-ditch response to stress, the third option when the more familiar fight-or-flight reaction proves impossible or ineffective. It is like playing possum—the animal appears to be dead—and in its altered state it is oblivious to pain. This also preserves one last chance for survival in case an opportunity for escape may yet arise, as it did for this lucky impala.

Even more amazing than this built-in survival mechanism was what happened afterward. The impala literally shook out the adrenaline-fueled energy that had built up during this near-death experience. And then it quickly returned to normal, looking as though this entire scenario had never happened. Wouldn't it be nice if we, too, could simply shake off the effects of our day-to-day traumas?

The fact is that we can. We all have the ability to discharge this excess energy and to reset ourselves back to our normal baseline. Research by Dr. Levine and others shows that even after severe trauma, self-corrective healing is possible.[1]

Fortunately, most of us never experience life-threatening trauma, but we all face less severe traumas, the daily stresses and perceived threats that nonetheless create a buildup of energy. The aftereffects of such stress reside in the body as physical tension and in the mind as worry or rumination. It is a generally unpleasant feeling that we call "being stressed" or "stressed out." The problem is that we seldom *do* discharge the energy, letting it build up so much that it may feel as if there is indeed a threat to our life. Vigorous movement, like the shaking of the impala, can discharge that energy. Daily exercise and even physical work can carry similar benefits for us.

It would be better, though, to release the energy of stress each day, perhaps multiple times per day, so that it doesn't even build up in the first place.

There is more to life than increasing its speed.

—GANDHI

Life is likely no more stressful now than it has ever been, but this may be the first time in history that stress has been so constant and unremitting. It is not natural or healthy to live such fast-paced lives, to be always "on," busy, or stressed. With regard to the stress response, the real problem lies in the failure to recover and reset back to baseline, and to do so regularly. Stress itself is not the issue so much as the inability to recover fully from it before the next stressful event occurs. If our lives are such that they are *always* stressful, then our bodies never get the chance to recover.

Observing nature reveals over and over again the importance of rhythms and cycles—basic life principles that we would do well to follow. There is a natural need for the body to cycle between activity and rest, movement and stillness. Life is not linear, though we try to make it so with constant productivity or continuous improvement. It ebbs and flows, and then does so again. Your own life may be enhanced if you learn to flow with it, to honor the restorative rhythms of rest and relaxation.

Why, then, don't we do it? Why is it that for so many of us, there is little to no time when we aren't *doing* something, when we fully free ourselves from our cell phones, computers, e-mail, voice mail—whatever it is that keeps us "wired"? Why is there so little downtime?

The reasons for this seem simple enough. First, our minds love to be distracted. It may be a means of escape from something in our lives that we don't want to face; it may be a way to avoid what we see as the unpleasantness of boredom; or it may simply be the untamed mind's default mechanism. Left to its own devices, the nature of the mind is to stay busy. The means we have available for distracting ourselves (such as Web surfing, video games, media, Facebook, Twitter, and the like) are alluring, even addicting. They are so powerful, and our minds are so distractible, that we must counter these tendencies intentionally. Few of us are able to live as sanely as baseball great Satchel Paige, who famously said, "Sometimes I sits and thinks, and sometimes I just sits." So if we don't give the mind a break on purpose, it is unlikely to happen.

Second, being busy is rewarded in our culture. Productivity is king, and we look up to those who are most "successful," who accomplish the most or make the most money. Those who excel in this way tend to be the most driven, the busiest, the best at multitasking. We don't honor those who are best at slowing down and enjoying the simple things in life.

We need to challenge our definition of success and the incessant busyness that it breeds. An unknown Chinese philosopher gives us another option: "The mark of a successful man is one who has spent an entire day on the bank of a river without feeling guilty about it."

The third reason: we simply forget. It may seem unnecessary to be reminded to do something that is good for us, and also easy, free, even enjoyable. But if we are not reminded constantly, most of us forget to stop doing things in order to give ourselves time to do nothing.

Apparently, this is not a new problem. Even in biblical times, people needed to be reminded, commanded even, to take a Sabbath day of rest. This included an aspect of devotion to the sacred, but part of its wisdom was simply to rest, to have a day each week without work. Many of us recall a time when there was one day a week when most stores were closed, there were no sporting events or other activities scheduled for kids, and hardly anyone worked. There may remain pockets of such a Sabbath tradition, but as a culture, we have all but given it away.

Being dormant, allowing for a period in which we lie fallow and restore ourselves, is good for us. In fact, when we are busiest or most stressed, we might gain the most from slowing down, stopping for a time, and resting. It may even make us more productive. As the Roman poet Ovid said, "Take rest; a field that has rested gives a bountiful crop."

Sometimes the cure for restlessness is rest.

—COLLEEN WAINWRIGHT

It is not difficult to rest or relax. Few instructions are required, because it is the simplest, most natural thing in the world. We only have to remember, and then allow ourselves to fall into a state of repose. The body will respond, if given a chance, and will set itself right. It will automatically recover from the effects of stress if allowed to do so. It is hungering for rest.

There are a few conditions that may facilitate this letting go into rest. It does, of course, require *time*—at least a few conscious moments sprinkled throughout the day. The less you feel bound by time, the less pressure you feel to squeeze in a little R & R, the more benefit you will receive from rest. Think of it more as an attitude toward life rather than one more thing to add to your to-do list.

If you like rituals, you may expand this time for recovery by beginning and ending with a simple act such as ringing a bell or lighting a candle. Like punctuation, this act sets the time apart from the rest of your day. Ritual can also add a sense of the sacred if you so choose.

Or you may find it helpful to choose something that you are likely to encounter during the day, such as a stoplight, a ringing phone, or the start of a meal, and use that as a reminder to let yourself relax. It could serve as your "mindfulness bell"—anything that occurs randomly throughout the day and serves to remind you to come back to awareness of the moment.

There is also a requirement of *space*. Again, it does not take much, but it may be helpful to think about creating a sense of openness and spaciousness around you. This could be as elaborate as finding a sanctuary that you go to, such as a beautiful worship space or a special garden or other outdoor area imbued for you with spirit. Or it could be as simple as having a small altar in the corner of a room, or even turning your office or your car into a sanctuary simply by intending it to be so for a few moments. You may also want to free yourself from some of the electronic entanglements that are so distracting to the mind. Try finding a place without computers or other screens, phones, or even doorbells. Or simply shut them off for a bit.

Intention is another of the requirements. After a time, relaxation may come so easily that you don't even need to think about it. But if you haven't done so for a long time, relaxation requires your willingness and intention. It is not something that can be forced to happen, any more than you can force yourself to fall asleep. You must be willing to let go, to relax into the moment.

And finally, there is *awareness*. If you place your awareness fully on any of the things listed below, you can give your mind a reprieve from its nonstop thinking and help both mind and body recover from stress. Another word to describe this kind of awareness is *mindfulness*.

You may think that you have to be practiced at meditation to be mindful, but you don't. There are other good things that can come from meditation, of course, as we will discuss in detail in the next few chapters. But being mindful—placing your awareness with intention from one moment to the next—is something natural that you already have the ability to do. You will get much better at it when the mind settles a bit, but start wherever you are and know that you have an in-nate capacity for mindful awareness that just needs a little attention to really blossom.

The rest of this chapter lists five opportunities for bringing more mindful, restorative rest into your life: breathing, sensing, walking, eating, and sleeping. Remember that this is not meant to give you more things to do. In fact, you already do each of them every day. It is more about the quality of presence that you bring as you are doing them. Or thinking of it another way, you are doing *nothing*—or at least not being productive—and still feeling good about it.

Breathe

Let's begin with one of nature's most basic cycles: the simple act of breathing in and breathing out. It is also one of the most commonly taught techniques for stress reduction—because it *works*. When people think of relaxation techniques, what often comes to mind is deep, abdominal breathing. In fact, research has shown it to be effective at inducing relaxation *and* improving performance.[2]

This practice is really simple, and you don't need to do anything to complicate it. You don't even have to breathe in any certain way. A study was done comparing various breathing instructions to see if one was better than another in terms of positively affecting physiology. They found that specific breathing instructions made little difference. What worked best was simply guiding participants to pay attention to breathing.[3]

In other words, don't try too hard. You don't need to breathe any certain way. Just pay attention to your breath, and it will naturally slow down and deepen, especially if you are able to relax your belly, allowing for more freedom of movement.

Mindfulness Practice: Breathing with Awareness

- You may sit, lie down, or even stand. Just try to be comfortable.
- Eyes may be open or closed. If it helps you to focus your attention, close them.
- Turn your attention toward your breath. Try to assume a beginner's mind, an attitude of interest and curiosity, as if you had never really noticed it before.
- Spend some time noticing every little nuance that you can: the coolness of the air as it enters the nostrils, the slight turbulence as it flows past the sinuses, the curving flow as it goes behind the throat, the entry into the large airways, the filling of the chest. Then notice everything in reverse as the breath is released.
- Place your attention anywhere you'd like: the back, chest, shoulders, or belly. In each place, you can experience the movement up and down, in and out, expanding and contracting.
- Ride the waves of the breath for a few cycles, rising and

falling, rising and falling, as though you were floating on top of the water in a warm ocean bay, being gently lifted and lowered by the swells of the waves.

- You do not need to change your breath in any way. Just notice it and let your belly soften, and the breath will slow and deepen of its own accord.

Awareness of breathing can be practiced for as long as you'd like. In just a few minutes a day you will become adept at it. Then you can follow the suggestion we make in our program. We encourage participants to do the Three Breaths Meditation, described below, several times per day. This is an incredibly easy way to create pauses throughout the day, requiring only as long as it takes to breathe three times.

To do the Three Breaths Meditation, whenever you think of it, place your attention on your breath for three full cycles. You can use your "mindfulness bell" as a trigger—remember that this can be anything of your choice, such as certain sounds (e.g., the phone ringing or the sound of an incoming e-mail) or events (the start of a meal, being stopped in traffic, having to wait in line). You may even wish to set the alarm on your cell phone to ring several times throughout the day to remind you to pause and pay deep attention to three breaths.

As you get better at it, you can even use the feeling of being stressed as your trigger to do the Three Breaths Meditation. Whenever you begin to feel bad—stressed out, anxious, angry, impatient—turn your attention toward your breathing. Three breaths, when done with awareness, may be all it takes to bring you back to yourself, to get you back on track and out of your thinking or unpleasant feeling. Try it— you may be surprised.

Sense

A few years ago I was biking in the southern Minnesota countryside on a perfect summer day. There were gently rolling hills, lush farm fields, and rustic barns in every direction. I was riding along a crest with all of this beauty before me when I became aware that I wasn't really seeing any of it. My mind was so preoccupied with some trouble, trying to figure it out by analyzing it for the hundredth time, that I couldn't see what I was looking at. My body was in the midst of beauty, but my mind was far, far away.

That was a moment of waking up for me. I realized all of a sudden that I wasn't really there, and knew that that was true for me most of the time. Just having that awareness helped bring me back into that moment's experience, though it's taken me a long time to become adept at doing so.

Now I know how simple it is—it just takes practice. Without realizing it, what I had been practicing for so long was thinking, analyzing, and being distracted. I had become very good at it. But with a little time and attention, it is equally possible to become good at being absorbed in the moment.

Your sensory experience, since it is so immediate and is often pleasurable, gives a perfect opportunity for developing this skill. With time, perhaps you will not miss your perfect summer days, the kind that Milan Kundera referred to when he wrote: "To sit with a dog on a hillside on a glorious afternoon is to be back in Eden, where doing nothing was not boring—it was peace."[4]

You can practice bringing attention to any of the senses. Here I describe listening to music, but you could just as easily listen to the sound of running water, or to singing birds, playing children, a breeze flowing through the trees. Or you could use any of the other senses—sight, touch, taste, smell. Anything that is available can be an invitation to awareness, even things that we might think are unpleasant, such as a noisy lawn mower or the sounds of traffic. But start with something you enjoy.

Mindfulness Practice: Listening with Awareness

- Choose one of your favorite sounds—perhaps something calming like classical music or sounds of nature.
- See to it that you won't be interrupted.
- Sit or lie down comfortably, eyes open or closed (if you can stay awake). If possible, surround yourself with the sound.
- Let go of all other thoughts or activities. Do nothing during this time but listen deeply.
- No matter how many times you have heard this before, approach it as if this is the first time, and this is the most interesting music you can imagine.
- As you listen, try not to think about or evaluate the sound. Let yourself absorb it. See if you can listen not just with the ears, but also with the whole body.
- Enjoy this awareness practice for as long and as often as you'd like.

Walk

I once had a meditation teacher whose first several years of mindfulness practice involved simply bringing awareness into her everyday routine. She was a single mother of three young children, had to work full-time, and had no time to sit down to meditate. So her meditation was walking mindfully from her bedroom to the children's rooms—just a few feet down the hallway. This didn't happen by chance—she had to intentionally bring her awareness into those brief walks. That is something you can do as well, and it is one of the most powerful mindfulness practices available.

You can choose to be more aware in any moment—bathing in the morning, cleaning the kitchen, stepping outside to get the mail, driving the car. How many times each day do you go from point A to point B without noticing anything in between? Try sometime to turn your errand or trip into an awareness exercise. Experiment with holding no agenda at all—just an intention to be present.

Mindfulness Practice: Walking with Awareness

- This may be incorporated into your daily activities, which often involve walking from here to there. However, try adding a time to walk when you don't have to get somewhere.
- Give yourself twenty to thirty minutes without trying to achieve anything—nowhere to go, nothing special to see, not even using it as exercise. Just walk for the pleasure of walking.
- If possible, go outdoors, preferably in a natural setting.
- Make it more of a stroll, noticing if you have a tendency to push the pace, and then consciously slowing down.
- Hold the intention to notice as much as you can: to sense the movement of your body, to feel the light touch of the air on your skin, to smell anything that is in the air, to see everything around you as deeply as you can.
- Be full of wonder—what will this moment bring? Notice what you are drawn to, and let your attention go there.
- When something catches your interest, let yourself linger

upon it for as long as you'd like. Smell the flowers, touch the stone, look deeply at the patterns in the sky. Remember, you have nowhere to go and nothing to do but to be fully where you are.

- Pay attention to your own sense of timing. When it feels right to stop and sense things, then stop. When you feel that it is time to move on, then move on.
- When your time is done, notice how you feel. Since there is no goal, you can't lose. However you feel is fine; whatever you have experienced is good.

Eat

Here is another opportunity for awareness, based upon an activity that most of us do several times a day—eating. It combines several aspects of mindfulness practice at once. There is the smell, taste, and feel of the food; the movement of the hands, tongue, and jaw; the pleasure inherent in eating good and healthy food; care of the self by the food choices we make; abundance in all the variety and quantity of food available to most of us. You can notice cravings, such as wanting more and more of a certain food or taste; or you may have aversions, disliking particular tastes and textures. You may notice the automatic tendency to eat quickly, mindlessly, or excessively; or the potential to sense when you have had enough and then choose to stop eating.

Among the benefits, this can be one way out of the trap of overeating and obesity. It can increase one's daily pleasure and help in making good food choices as you try to eat more brain-healing foods. Try to do this practice of mindful eating every so often, and then think about ways to bring this type of awareness into other everyday activities.

Mindfulness Practice: Eating with Awareness

- Set aside a mealtime to eat alone or in silence with others.
- Put some thought into what you want to eat. Choose healthy, wholesome, and flavorful fare.
- Prepare the food with awareness and attention.
- Sit down, close your eyes, and allow the mind to quiet for a few moments.
- Give thanks for your food. Gratitude connects you to the fabric of life and is as nourishing as any single aspect of the food.
- Look at the food, the shape and color and amount of it.
- Before you take your first bite, notice the feeling of hunger in the belly, the sense of anticipation, the changes in your mouth as it prepares to receive the food.
- Smell it before putting it in your mouth. Feel the warmth, substance, and texture as you touch it to the lips and then place it in the mouth. Taste each bite, noticing how different the experience of taste is in different areas of the mouth.
- Pay special attention to that first bite, how vividly you taste it, how the tongue and entire mouth come alive.
- Chew each bite slowly, resisting the urge to swallow quickly and move on to the next bite. Make each bite a deliberate act, one to be savored and enjoyed.
- Pay attention to the mechanics of eating, the movement of jaw and tongue, the way your body knows how to handle the food, chewing and moving it back toward the throat.
- Keep some of your awareness on your stomach, noticing especially when you are beginning to feel satisfied, as though you have had enough. See if you can stop eating before you have the sensation of fullness.

- Try to do this for at least part of each meal, and do it for
  an entire meal as often as you can.

Sleep

At the very start of this book I told the story of Catherine, whose recent discovery of cancer had sent her into a tailspin. Her mind was spinning out of control, and though her cancer had been successfully treated, she was greatly concerned about her degree of anxiety. I felt sure that the central problem was her inability to sleep. "If you can get some sleep," I reassured her, "I'm confident that you'll feel a whole lot better within a few days." That turned out to be true.

How could I be so sure that dealing with sleep would turn things around for Catherine? Because after practicing for nearly twenty-five years and seeing thousands of patients, I have come to appreciate the truth of this statement by Thomas Dekker, a seventeenth-century English poet: "[Sleep is] the golden chain that ties health and our bodies together."[5]

Trouble sleeping is the most common trigger for an episode of anxiety, depression, or even more severe mental illness. Stress may have caused the sleep problem, but it is often inadequate sleep that tips us into illness. If we aren't sleeping, the body cannot effectively turn off the stress response.[6]

The opposite is also true. Sleeping well may lead to a quick recovery, and improving sleep is often the only intervention needed if it is done early enough. With two or three good nights' sleep, we may feel more balanced and more like ourselves almost immediately. That is what happened for Catherine, even though she had been struggling with her symptoms, and insomnia, for weeks.

Problems with sleep affect fifty to seventy million Americans.[7]

The most common problem is sleep deprivation—we simply don't get enough sleep. If you are like most people, you need about one hour more than you are getting each night. Most adults need approximately seven to eight hours per night but are only getting six to seven hours. Much of that is due to lifestyle—we just don't allow ourselves enough time for sleep.

If you are often tired or sleepy during the day, if you require an alarm every day and still struggle to get up in the morning, or if you want to nap frequently (whether or not you actually nap), then you, too, are not getting enough sleep.

One of the difficulties with sleep is that it cannot be forced. You cannot *make* yourself fall asleep, and the harder you try or the worse you want it, the harder it can become to get it. But while you cannot control when you fall asleep, you can usually control when you awaken. If you arise at a consistent time, you will soon be able to fall asleep more easily and naturally. Try the following experiment to determine your personal sleep needs.

Finding Your True Sleep Number: How Many Hours Do You Need?

- Choose a wake-up time that you can live with—preferably between six and eight in the morning. Get up within an hour of that time *every* day (even on weekends).
- See if you can stretch out your nights by gradually allowing yourself an earlier bedtime. Go to bed about fifteen minutes earlier each night until you wake at your desired time without an alarm.

- Keep yourself to that schedule for at least two or three weeks. When you consistently wake refreshed without an alarm, you've discovered the amount of sleep you really need.
- Note that your natural sleep amount may change over the course of the year—most need less in the summer and more in the winter. Allow yourself to change, within limits, with the seasons.
- Aim for seven to nine hours per night throughout the year, and keep your wake-up time consistent.

Most of us are voluntarily sleep-deprived, but there are also millions of Americans with insomnia—that is, they *can't* sleep. Nearly everyone encounters this problem occasionally, but for many people insomnia becomes a chronic problem lasting weeks, months, even years.

In our Resilience Training Program, we find that most participants suffer from chronic insomnia. And though treating insomnia is not a central part of the program, nearly everyone's sleep improves. According to our early data, the average amount of sleep increases from five hours to seven hours per night by the end of the program. I believe this is one of the main reasons people feel so much better.

Here is the advice that I share with the participants for getting a good night's sleep. There are three common patterns to insomnia:

1. Trouble falling asleep
2. Waking in the middle of the night
3. Waking too early in the morning

We will look at these separately, and I will offer natural solutions for each problem. For more information about the supplements, including dosage, you may refer back to chapter 5.

"I Can't Fall Asleep"

Known as "initial insomnia," having trouble falling asleep is the most common pattern of sleep disturbance and is usually caused by one of three things:

Stress/Anxiety

This is the problem most everyone is familiar with. When you go through a stressful time, you go to bed but your mind kicks in and you can't stop thinking—often worrying, fearing the future or trying to figure things out.

Natural Solutions

- Practice awareness-of-breath meditation shortly before bed.
- Use a calming herb such as valerian, passionflower, or chamomile, or an amino acid such as tryptophan, L-theanine or GABA.

Disrupted Biorhythms Due to Getting Up at Irregular Times

If you allow yourself to sleep in by more than an hour in the morning, your body may not be ready for sleep at the usual time the following night. This is a really common problem for young people, but as we age we become even more sensitive to these circadian rhythm changes.

Natural Solutions

- Get up at about the same time every day. Try not to sleep in by more than an hour, even on weekends.
- Occasionally use melatonin until you are back on

schedule. I prefer using sublingual melatonin, as it is absorbed more quickly and goes directly to where it is needed. A dose of 2–3 mg just before bedtime is usually sufficient.

Overstimulation

You can be overstimulated by a substance such as caffeine or a decongestant, for example, or by stimulating activities done too close to bedtime. Use of electronic media, intense conversations, performing busywork or frustrating tasks, and even exercise done too close to bedtime may raise the tone of the nervous system.

Natural Solutions

- Stop stimulating activities at least thirty to sixty minutes before bed. Replace them with something soothing or calming, such as reading, gentle stretching, or meditation.
- Avoid taking decongestants late in the day. These are found in many antihistamines and cold remedies. Look for pseudoephedrine or phenylephrine on the label, or the letter D after the brand name (e.g., Claritin-D).
- Gradually reduce caffeine until you no longer have trouble falling asleep. You may not even be able to drink it in the morning until sleep improves.

"I Can't Stay Asleep"

Waking in the middle of the night (middle insomnia) is often due to one of these common problems:

Stress

Elevated cortisol can result in light, easily disrupted sleep.

Natural Solutions

- Most of the practices in the Resilience Training Program are helpful at dampening the stress response. Exercise is especially good for middle insomnia.
- It's easier to sleep when the body is cool. Exercise at least two hours prior to bedtime if possible, so that your body has time to cool off.
- Likewise, if you bathe at night, finish an hour or so before bed.

Antidepressants

Prozac and other SSRIs often cause middle insomnia.

Natural Solutions

- If taking an SSRI for depression or anxiety and middle insomnia is a problem, talk with your doctor about changing the timing or dosage, or adding something to reduce this problem. If the medication is new to you, sleep may improve in a few weeks.

Alcohol

Consuming alcohol, especially two or more drinks, shortly before bed can cause middle insomnia. It is common to awaken as the alcohol's effects wear off.

Natural Solutions

- Limit yourself to a small drink earlier in the evening, perhaps with supper. Better yet, don't drink at all until your sleep is normal.

Eating Too Much or Too Little Before Bed

If you eat a large amount or have a fatty snack, the digestive system has to work too hard to allow for good rest. Low blood sugar, caused by too few calories in the evening, or a high-sugar snack just before bed sends alarm bells to the brain, also disrupting sleep.

Natural Solutions

- Try to have supper early in the evening. If you have to eat later, make it a small meal. Do not go to bed hungry, though, and if supper has been more than 3 hours before bedtime, have a modest snack of a low-glycemic carbohydrate, like a whole grain. A small amount of healthy fat can also help, but avoid large amounts of protein or fat at bedtime.

Having to Urinate

You may need to get up in the night, disrupting your sleep pattern, if you drink too many fluids in the evening.

Natural Solutions

- Limit fluids in the evening, even during supper.

"I Wake Up Too Early and Can't Fall Back to Sleep"

Waking too early in the morning (terminal insomnia) may be a result of several things.

Use of Short-Acting Sedatives

Sleeping medication, alcohol, or even melatonin—things we take to help us sleep—sometimes can actually cause terminal insomnia. Sometimes when they wear off, there is a rebound to a more alert state.

Natural Solutions

- Avoid short-acting sedatives if possible. Even some of the popular sleep medications wear off too early.

Depression

When related to depression, early waking is a reflection of abnormal adrenal (stress) hormones. The body loses the ability to shut down the adrenal gland, resulting in getting a natural wake-up call too early.

Natural Solutions

- Try herbs such as St. John's wort, valerian, or passion-flower, or amino acids such as L-theanine or 5-HTP. Refer to *The Chemistry of Joy* for a complete natural approach to depression.

General Stress

Terminal insomnia can also be due to general stress, which elevates cortisol levels, lightens sleep, and reduces the length of the sleep cycle.

Natural Solutions

- Try any of the supplements listed in chapter 5 for toning down the stress response. Long-acting supplements, such as passionflower or L-theanine, have a better chance of remaining effective through the night. Products that combine several substances may work best.
- If you find you're quite hungry upon waking, have a larger snack at bedtime.

The practices in this chapter offer a chance to calm the number one obstacle to peace: your own mind. As you tame your mind, it will be easier to relax and restore yourself. The two effects are mutually reinforcing. We will work more directly with the thinking mind, and learn how to settle it, in the next chapter.

PART TWO

Awaken to Equanimity

8

Step 4: Quiet the Mind

Why Mindfulness Is the Key to Restoring Your Calm

We live in a flash of light; evening comes and it is night forever. It's only a flash and we waste it. We waste it with our anxiety, our worries, our concerns, our burdens.

—ANTHONY DE MELLO

Key Points

- While there are external sources of pain and stress in our lives, it is our own mind that creates worry, anxiety, and much of our unnecessary suffering.
- We give power to that which we give attention, and anxious thoughts have too much influence. Without questioning them, we believe our thoughts to be true.
- Mindfulness practice provides an antidote to the unsettled mind. It helps us to refine skills we already possess but which may be hidden: a steady mind, focused attention, the ability to explore and reflect on our experiences without judging them—or ourselves— too harshly.

THE RESILIENCE Training Program is founded on the belief that you are fundamentally healthy, but that something has gotten in the way of that natural health to create what is often considered "disease." Resilience implies that it is possible to bounce back, to recover that which has been obscured or taken away. Even if illness has been there for a very long time, health can always be reclaimed. It is still there, waiting to be reawakened.

Many believe that there is some sort of mystery to good mental health that can put it just beyond our reach. That is untrue. There are self-righting skills that can be learned by anyone with the desire and motivation to do so. The path that we will take toward these skills is what I call the "psychology of mindfulness."

Mindfulness consists largely of learning to pay attention to our experience with minimal input from the judging nature of the mind. We all have had experiences of mindfulness and have the capacity to take in the fullness of the moment. We have had that ability since early childhood. But there are so many competing forces, and so little encouragement to support those skills, that for the vast majority of us they have atrophied. We must reclaim and strengthen our inherent ability to remain present in each moment.

If you have suffered with intense anxiety or depression, this may sound like a frightening possibility; being fully present sometimes feels intolerable. Still, becoming more skillful with our minds and emotions is the most reliable way to reclaim resilience and happiness. The gateway to resilience is our capacity to be present.

The Source of Our Discontent

Mindfulness comes out of the Buddhist tradition, which has a great deal to say about the nature of suffering. The Four Noble Truths, which form the foundation of the Buddha's teachings, all refer to suffering and the pathway out of it. To live is to suffer—pain and loss are unavoidable. Beyond the unavoidable, however, there is a nearly constant sense of dissatisfaction, feeling unhappy or discontent with the way things are. We weave back and forth between desire and distaste, between pleasure and displeasure, trying to find that razor's edge where things are "just right." But even when we achieve that sense of satisfaction, it doesn't last. We veer off one way or the other—we seek more of something we like, or try to avoid something we don't like. Either way, we are not happy with how things are in that moment.

Oftentimes we cannot change what is. But we fail to recognize that the feeling of discontent comes not from the circumstances outside of ourselves but from our own wish that things were different from how they are. It is our *attachment* to wanting things to be a certain way, and frustration when they are not, that makes us feel so bad. It is our thinking mind that causes our discontent.

Since we don't recognize that the primary source of our dissatisfaction lies within, we continue to believe that there is something just outside our grasp that would make us happy if we could only attain it: "If only I had a nicer car . . . a better job . . . a more understanding spouse—then I would be content." Or instead of pulling things toward ourselves, perhaps we are pushing them away: "I wish I didn't have to write this report . . . hadn't lost so much money in the stock market . . . didn't have to deal with anxiety every day—then I wouldn't feel so unhappy." If we don't like our experience as it is, we wish that we could escape it.

You may recall the arrow metaphor from chapter 1. There are wounds that we receive in life that are unavoidable and not of our own making: physical pain, loss of a loved one, betrayal by a friend or lover, failure to achieve what we set out to do. Those are the "first arrows," and everyone experiences them.

But on top of those painful experiences we add layer upon layer of optional suffering. These wounds are largely self-inflicted by a mind that is not yet able to recognize what it is doing—hurting oneself with the unnecessary "second arrows" of thought, grasping for what it thinks is missing, or rejecting what is painful. This discontent often leads to a great deal of wasted energy in a futile effort to change what is. Yet that effort only creates further distress—and on and on the cycle goes.

Let me share a personal example of how the mind can create unnecessary suffering. Several years ago, early in the month of April, I was sitting by a window—meditating, actually—in my home in Minneapolis. I distinctly remember seeing how dreary and unpleasant everything looked at that time of year. I noticed the drab colors, the power lines visible between the houses, the closeness of the older homes with no foliage to hide their blemishes. Everything around me seemed unattractive and unappealing.

As I sat there, I was aware only that I was unhappy. I didn't realize that the source of my unhappiness, in that moment, lay primarily with my perceptions and judgments, creations of my own mind. Not knowing any better, I began looking for external reasons why I felt unhappy—and it was very easy to find them: *It's this dilapidated old house in this lousy, run-down neighborhood. I don't like my job, and we live in this big city where everyone is so busy and disconnected.*

These thoughts had an unsettling effect upon me, leaving me feeling restless and a little agitated. I arose from my meditation to find my wife, so that I could share my "insights" with her. I even walked around the house with her to point out all of the things that were wrong with it.

It didn't stop there. I thought that since there was an external problem, there must also be an external solution. *We need to move to a smaller town, live in a nicer neighborhood, find a job that keeps me in the community. My life will be so much more integrated. Then I'll be happy.*

As I kept repeating these thoughts, I came to believe them. Soon I believed them so much that I mobilized all kinds of energy to change things. I convinced my wife, who didn't want to move, that we should follow my plan. Within four months, we had sold our house, bought a new one, packed up the kids, and moved the entire family to a small town nearby where I found a job with a local medical group.

I didn't realize until much later that my unhappiness came from within myself. I wasn't aware that my mind at that moment of discontent was scanning, looking for the source of my unhappiness. I took those simple thoughts and rehearsed and magnified them until I believed them to be true. And they generated so much power that I left a job that I had previously loved, moved out of an older but lovely prairie-style home, and left a community of friends and colleagues that I had spent five years cultivating.

That is not to say that it was a mistake, either. It turned out to be a great move for the family and I've ended up in a wonderful place professionally. But it led to a very painful and unnecessary set of transitions that left me struggling for a number of years. At the time, I didn't know how to do it differently. I didn't yet realize the degree to which I had given my life over to my own thoughts and feelings.

It didn't occur to me that I would take my thinking with me when I moved to another city. Though I had heard it before, I didn't fully understand that freedom comes from within. I had not yet learned the practical skills that can give you that freedom from the tyranny of an untamed mind.

The Power of Thought

This is no small force, the power inherent in our minds. As an example, consider these comments made by Larry Summers, economic advisor to President Obama, taken from a speech about the White House's response to the economic crisis. The date was March 13, 2009—a time of great fear and uncertainty, as the nation and the world appeared to be tumbling toward a complete economic meltdown. He was speaking about the rare circumstances we were in, when the normally self-correcting forces in the market became "overwhelmed by vicious cycles."

> Greed gives way to fear. And this fear begets fear.
>
> This is the paradox at the heart of the financial crisis. In the past few years, we've seen too much greed and too little fear; too much spending and not enough saving; too much borrowing and not enough worrying. Today, however, our problem is exactly the opposite.
>
> It is this transition from an excess of greed to an excess of fear that President Roosevelt had in mind when he famously observed that the only thing we had to fear was fear itself. It is this transition that has happened in the United States today.

Dr. Summers suggested that there had not been *enough* worrying prior to this meltdown. He is rightly pointing to the positive aspects of paying attention, being thoughtful and aware. By showing greater care and foresight, perhaps we could have avoided this crisis. But he is also saying that these forces, powerful enough to bring a great economy to its knees, are largely in our collective minds.

One reason it is so hard to break out of the cycle of habitual thought is because almost everyone else is caught up in it, too. We have built a consensus reality, where nearly everyone implicitly agrees to believe in his or her thoughts. Like you, most of the rest of us are empowering his or her own thoughts without realizing that we are doing so. Fear begets fear. Fearful thinking is contagious, and when enough people share in such a belief, it may become the very "truth" that we fear.

The Nature of Mind

The above examples show how unexamined thoughts can become painful reality, on both the personal and societal levels. But it doesn't have to happen that way.

What is missing in both of these examples is *awareness*. Without awareness that thoughts are just thoughts, the mind automatically makes them appear real. When we are aware that we are thinking, we can see thoughts for what they are, question their validity, reflect upon them, and choose whether or not to believe them or act upon them.

So why would we do this to ourselves? Why would we harm ourselves with our own thinking if it was truly optional? Why wouldn't we simply add awareness and spare ourselves this unnecessary pain?

Pema Chodron gives a very straightforward explanation for this: "Because you have been training in wild mind. You started as a baby with a little bit of it, and you've just been getting better and better at it as you get older."[1]

Since childhood we have spent many of our waking hours reinforcing our habits of thought. We empower them through attention and repetition. Anything that we practice this consistently we will eventually get good at.

However, this "wild mind" is not the end of the story. It's not even the *beginning* of the story. We all began life with a more open, expansive mind, one that was naturally able to be fully present in the moment. Observe young children and you will see the truth of that. They are awake, they see things with fresh eyes, and their minds are flexible and open. This is the *natural mind*, still present in each of us even though it may be obscured by thought. And it remains available to us in each moment, if we know how to access it.

"Your mind and my mind are no different than the mind of the most awakened," adds Pema Chodron. "It's just that we don't recognize the true nature of mind, and we identify more with the craziness, the wildness."[2]

The true nature of the mind is like a blue sky on a sunny day— open, clear, and expansive. When we are in our "natural mind," thinking seems effortless, creative thoughts arise spontaneously, we work efficiently, and we are able to play with equal ease. But when we get caught up in the turbulence of our thinking, it is as if clouds have moved in overhead. The vast openness is still there beyond the clouds, but from our vantage point on the ground we lose sight of it.

Still, the clear openness remains available to us in any moment, even during the storms. The difference between one who is "awakened" and the majority of us who are not is that we don't realize that the clouds are just temporary manifestations of our own thinking. We become identified with our thoughts and forget that it is we who are generating them. And if the clouds remain for a long time, it is easy to forget that the sun exists at all. The awakened ones remember that, and know that they can connect with the openness under any circumstances, at any moment. We can learn to do that, too.

Settling the Mind

"I'm an anxious person in general," Jeannie said. "I have been since high school, if not before." She is now in her mid-forties, and anxiety has impacted everything in her life, including her career, marriage, and parenting. While she was in graduate school she had her first full-blown panic attacks. She felt so stressed out by school that she took a full year off, worked with a therapist, and slowly recovered. But when she tried to return, another severe panic episode derailed her schooling entirely, leaving her with a sense of despair and the fear that she would never be able to support herself. This time, therapy did not seem to help.

At that point she turned to medication, and it worked like a miracle at first. "I cried in relief at how much better I felt," she said. But that was sixteen years ago, and since then medications have become less and less effective. They have also caused numerous side effects—nagging problems that she would have gladly put up with if the medication had kept working for her. But after trying many different medications, she finally gave up on them the year before she saw me. She came to the Resilience Training Program hoping for a different approach. "I just want to learn something I can do for myself."

Jeannie was already careful with her diet and diligent about exercising. She began the basic supplement program, along with several additional supplements to improve sleep and calm her stress response. These measures helped a great deal but did not change the fundamental pattern of her thinking. That appeared to be the missing link in her recovery.

Like many people with long-term anxiety, Jeannie hadn't a clue as to how to work with her mind. So we began very simply, with awareness of breathing, just as we discussed in the last chapter. At first it felt nearly intolerable to her. "My mind is racing at a hundred miles an hour! I get so restless—after a couple of minutes, I can hardly stand it."

I encouraged her to stay with it. "Just sit for five minutes. If you can't sit any longer, then it's okay to get up and do a walking meditation. But try to keep the focus on your breath. If you can do it even for three breaths, it will help your mind settle down."

Jeannie was so motivated to change that she *did* stay with it. She learned to tolerate her restlessness and remain still, at least in body.

She slowly became better at keeping her mind focused on her breath. "If you can learn to stay with your breath," I added, "you'll be able to focus on your thoughts. And that will help you tame them."

Identify with the Observer

When practicing mindfulness, we wish to connect with the blue-sky openness of the natural mind. One aspect of that larger mind is referred to as the "observing self." It is the part of us that remains above the fray, that doesn't get caught up in all of the drama contained in our thoughts. It is the aspect of our mind that remains calm and continues to see things more objectively, as they really are, and not through the distorted lens of perception or desire.

One of the phenomena that can be observed is the act of thinking itself. Seeing the workings of the mind as they are, in real time, allows us to separate ourselves from our thoughts rather than identify so closely with them.

If you have never knowingly had the experience of watching your thoughts, it may at first seem to make no sense. It is a bit like riding a bike—before you experience it for the first time, you may not get it at all, but once you have done it, even briefly, you implicitly understand what it means and how to do it. You may still need practice to become good at it, but you *get* it.

Here are the instructions for observing thought that I gave to Jeannie and the others in the class during our formal meditation practice.

Mindfulness Practice: Observing the Stream of Thought

Picture yourself sitting calmly on a riverbank, watching the water as it flows by. The river is your stream of consciousness. Thoughts come along, like something floating in the water. Your observing self is the one sitting alongside the river watching these thoughts come and go. Know that there is a part of you that is able to do this—to remain separate from your thoughts and unaffected by them, just sitting and watching them as they pass by.

Sometimes the mind is really turbulent, like a raging river churning with such activity that you can't make out one thought from the other. Just stay with your breath and allow the mind to settle if you can. Then go back to watching the stream of thought.

Other times the mind seems blank. It is as if the water is barely moving and there are no thoughts at all. If so, just enjoy the peacefulness. You don't have to try to generate thoughts. Eventually they will come on their own.

As you sit, try to notice an individual thought arise, as though it was carried from upstream and then appears before you. See if you can keep observing it as it passes in front of you and eventually disappears downstream. Soon another object presents itself to you. Your job is just to sit on the riverbank and observe. There is nothing you need to do, nothing you need to change.

Notice the different qualities of your thoughts. Some are very routine, even dull. Many you have had before, and some are replayed frequently. You may find yourself feeling bored by such mundane thoughts, so much that your energy falls or your awareness drops off. Do your best to remain present and attentive.

Occasionally a thought will come along that seems really interesting or important, and you will find yourself being drawn into it. Just remain calm and observe, without getting too caught up by the content. *Oh, there's a thought coming and going. Oh! There's another thought.*

Still other thoughts might be so compelling that you give up your seat on the riverbank and go into the stream, letting yourself get carried away by them. You may lose touch with your observing self and become absent for a few moments. As soon as you realize that you have done this, return to your seat on the riverbank and go back to observing your thoughts—without judging yourself for the lapse. Each time you remember to come back you are strengthening your mindfulness muscles.

Notice that each thought lasts just a short time, so long as you don't entertain it. It simply passes by the screen of your awareness. Eventually the thought fades, and then is replaced by another. This is repeated over and over again—for all of us.

The Power of Repetition

As Jeannie learned to observe her own thinking, she was shocked to see how often she repeated the same thoughts. At first, any given thought had little hold on her—it was just an idle thought that popped up, seemingly out of nowhere. But as she repeated that thought, she noticed herself starting to believe it to be true.

"If you give a thought 'airtime' in your mind, then you empower it," I explained. "This is similar to the role of a radio DJ, who helps create a hit song by playing it over and over again. The more you 'listen' to a favorite thought, reinforce it through repetition, the more it is strengthened. Soon you make it appear to be true by believing in it."

That is just as true for positive, loving thoughts as it is for negative or judging ones. Positive thoughts, too, can be reinforced through practice. We'll get to that later. But let's begin where you are—where almost all of us are. We create much of our suffering through our own thinking. We have to realize that we do this by seeing it in action before we can stop doing it.

To say that the mind is the primary source of suffering is not to deny that there are valid causes of pain and loss. Indeed, Jeannie had experienced a great deal of loss, much of it a result of her disabling anxiety. It is important to acknowledge this and to change any painful aspect of your life that you can. But the way to break the stress cycle is to stop struggling against your experience and learn to relate to it in new ways, to see and accept whatever is true without judgment, contraction, or pushing away.

Seeing Thoughts as Thoughts

Jeannie began to see what her mind was doing during 99 percent of her waking hours—it was generating thoughts, many of them based upon fears of the future or the belief that she was somehow flawed. As she realized the extent to which her own thoughts were affecting her, bringing her down and fueling her stress, she became discouraged. "What's wrong with me? Why do I think so many unhealthy thoughts?"

"Don't be hard on yourself," I responded. "You do this because you have a mind just like everyone else. This is just what the mind does—it creates thoughts. The thoughts themselves are neither good nor bad. They are just fleeting creations of the mind, and they will quickly pass away if you let them. The trick lies in seeing them for what they are—*they are just thoughts!* They aren't reality."

When you have the insight that the mind is generating thoughts, and they are *only* thoughts, then you can choose what to do with them. Jeannie, for example, frequently had this thought: *I can't get a good job, and if I do I won't keep it. How will I make a living? I'm not going to be able to support myself or my family.* Her mind generated these thoughts out of such long habit that she automatically believed them to be true—she didn't even question them.

She first recognized these as thoughts during her meditation practice, and with guidance she began to challenge them. "Thoughts will have their brief time in the spotlight, but don't keep them there by giving them your attention," I said. "Let them recede by declining to entertain them. Don't give them life by believing the content of the thoughts. Allow them to fall away simply by seeing that they are not True with a capital *T*."

With time, Jeannie began to absorb these lessons. Then she was able to reap the harvest of mindfulness practice by taking her new insights out into the rest of her life. With mindfulness as her ally, she could see similar thoughts arising during the course of her day. Then, in the difficult moments, she was able to recognize them as just thoughts, that's all. When she didn't react too strongly to them, when she gave them their allotted airtime but no more, they quickly faded and they lost their power over her.

Jeannie was thrilled with her progress. She began to identify more with her observing mind and less with her thinking mind. She understood that she had given away much of her power to her thoughts, but she was beginning to reclaim that power. "I can see that I am not my thoughts. I know how to recognize a thought for what it is and not just believe that it's true. When I do that, it seems to let the air out of it. The thought loses its punch."

Raising the Level of Awareness

It *is* as simple as that. You don't have to get inside your brain and work with each thought one by one. You only have to recognize what you are doing, see thoughts as thoughts, and let it go. When you raise your level of understanding about the process of thinking, you don't have to concern yourself with each individual thought.

Jeannie remained troubled by this. "If I'm really freeing myself up from the thinking mind, shouldn't I stop having these anxious thoughts? I thought the point was to get rid of them."

"Lots of luck," I said. "You cannot stop yourself from having particular thoughts, and if you try, you're likely to have even more of them. Thoughts come from who knows where, and when they fade they go back to who knows where. You cannot stop the process of thinking, and you can't stop certain thoughts from arising. So don't concern yourself with that. With time, you may find that your mind calms down so that you have fewer negative thoughts. But don't be alarmed if they still come back.

"You do, however, have the power to choose what to do after a thought has arisen, and you can prevent yourself from being harmed by your thoughts—so long as you remain aware. Your leverage is in the moment, while the thought is on the screen of your awareness. That's why you want to practice getting good at moment-to-moment awareness. It's all you have."

Learning to stay present to whatever is occurring in the moment is what is meant by *mindfulness practice*. The place that we can reduce our painful habits is within our own minds and hearts. The time that we can reclaim our freedom is in the present moment. It is in learning to be aware and fully alive to the moment, with all of its beauty and terror, that we can transform ourselves.

Mindfulness Meditation: Training for the Difficult Moments

Mindfulness is the energy of being aware and awake to the present moment. It is the continuous practice of touching life deeply in every moment of daily life. To be mindful is to be truly alive, present, and at one with those around you and with what you are doing.

—THICH NHAT HANH

Meditation is our training ground. It is where we build skills, presence, the capacity for courage, the ability to exercise choice. In the time spent sitting, attending to the body, breath, or mind, we will be confronted with all the experiences that happen in our larger lives outside of the meditation time. It is a microcosm for our lives. Our minds will see to it that everything comes before us—pain, joy, boredom, restlessness, memories, analyses, plans, contentment, wanting, aversion, falling asleep. It all happens in the safety of the meditation space, giving us the opportunity to practice how we respond so that, when we really need it, we have the presence of mind to deal with life in the healthiest way possible.

Since there is no particular goal or achievement inherent in this process, you are free to have whatever experience comes up for you. Try to hold on to the notion that whatever happens is okay and can be observed and learned from. There will be times when you feel deeply relaxed and other times when you are so restless you wonder why anyone would bother with this. At times you may feel real contentment, at other times boredom. Pain may come up, or difficult emotions, or memories, or great ideas or insights. For all of this, try to stay in touch with your observing self, not placing judgments on what comes up or on yourself for having the experiences. Just observe and learn, much like a scientist might do while studying animals in the wild—filled with curiosity, wonder, and awe.

When one first begins a consciousness practice of this sort, it may seem impossibly daunting. That may be especially true if you have suffered from chronic anxiety or depression, because one of the false beliefs is that *you* are not capable of change, even if others are. It is vitally important to plant the seed of a new belief: *it is at least possible to escape lifelong mental habits*. It is not possible to end all stress or suffering, but we all can, with some guidance and effort, reduce our unconscious tendency to make our suffering worse than it needs to be.

"There is nothing magical or special about these skills," I explained to Jeannie. "Everyone already has the inherent qualities and abilities to learn and practice this. Yes, you do create distress through your own thinking. But you also have the capacity to be calm and focused upon whatever you choose, without getting lost in thought."

There is no goal in meditation—yet it can give you the kind of insight and self-understanding that you cannot get in any other way. It is important to have direct experience through a personal practice in order to really learn and adopt these skills. Otherwise, it's like trying to learn to play a musical instrument just by listening to someone talk about it. You might understand it on an intellectual level, but only by picking up the instrument and practicing it do you really get it.

This is a practice filled with paradox. There is nothing to achieve, yet you set out to free yourself from the second arrow of harmful, habitual thought. You need strong intention and motivation, yet the serenity that you seek cannot be found through effort—in fact, effort may make it more elusive. It is not necessary to try so hard, because your clear mind has always been there; it has just been hidden by thought. All that is required is for you to realize that, and then you can return to your natural, calm mind. You can awaken to this reality in any given moment—but you have to do so *again and again*.

Mindfulness Practice: Meditation with Awareness of Thoughts

- Sit as comfortably as you can, back upright but not rigid. Hold yourself with dignity, as if you were royally born.
- Allow your eyes to close, or if you prefer, hold your gaze softly upon the floor or an object a few feet in front of you.
- Breathe through your nostrils. Sense the flow of the air as it passes the sinuses. Follow it into the lungs, feeling the chest expand. Allow the belly to be soft so that your breathing is naturally deep.

- Notice the very end point of your in-breath. Try to experience the moment that the tide turns and the in-breath has ended, but the out-breath has not yet begun. Then follow the breath all the way out as it passes through the chest, airways, and finally the nostrils. Notice how it is warmer and feels different as it leaves—the air has been transformed.

- Experience the moment when all the breath that is going to leave has done so, and the tide turns again. Then follow the next in-breath in the same way as before.

- Sit with awareness of breathing for a few more cycles—in and out, up and down, rising and falling.

- During the rest of the meditation, your breath can serve as your anchor. Whenever you notice that you have drifted off or lost touch with the moment, return to awareness of breathing for a few cycles to get back into your body, grounded again in the moment.

- Now allow your awareness to expand beyond the breath to include the rest of the body. Let yourself be drawn to any sensation that seems to be calling to you—the feel of your body sinking into the chair or cushion, the sense of being upheld, the warmth of your hands resting upon your lap, the slight coolness of the air on your skin.

- Notice if you have any discomfort in your body. Try to calmly observe the feeling of discomfort, allowing yourself to experience it for at least a short while without needing to change it. Then move if you'd like in order to make yourself more comfortable.

- Next, turn your attention outward from your body, noticing any sounds around you: subtle noises in the room, like a fan or the shuffling of others; outdoor sounds like wind or traffic; running water or singing birds, if you are in a natural setting. Just allow yourself to take in these sounds, with no need to change them in any way.

- Now invite your awareness to turn toward your mind and observe your own thinking. You might first notice the general quality of the mind: in this moment, is it active or still, turbulent or calm, generating a lot of thought or rather empty of thought? There is no need to wish it were different—simply notice it as it is.

- Sitting beside the stream of your awareness, calmly observe your thoughts. Try to notice a thought arise, watch it play across the screen of your awareness, and then allow it to fade away. Be aware of thoughts that seem to "stick," to grab your awareness or to change how you feel. Again, you don't need to change them—just observe them.

- After a time, you may find that you are no longer present to your experience. Your awareness may have faded, or perhaps you have been captured by your thoughts and carried away down the stream. No matter—as soon as you become aware again, let go of those particular thoughts and return to sitting and observing the stream of thought. Use your breath, if needed, to help bring you back to greater awareness in the moment.

- As you continue to sit in this way, you may feel as if your mind is constantly jumping around, or that you are repeatedly losing touch with the moment. It is okay—this is what the mind does. But each time you notice that it has happened, bring yourself back, without judgment of yourself, and with no need to wish it were different.

- You may notice an endless array of thoughts, or you may find that you repeat the same few thoughts over and over. Some thoughts are appealing, others distressing.

Remember that you do not need to change any of it—you only need to notice it. With time and acceptance, your thinking mind will change itself.

- Sit in this way for twenty to thirty minutes. At the end of this time, return your awareness to your breath. Allow yourself a few moments of feeling grateful to yourself for giving this kind of time and attention to your own mind. Accept the experience just as it has been.

When you begin a mindfulness practice you may find, as Jeannie did, that your mind is almost unbearably active and your body so restless that it is hard to remain still. But as you continue this practice, your mind has a chance to quiet itself, and the restlessness of the body tends to fade over time. You may also be surprised, when you see the nature of your thoughts up close and personal, to discover how many of them are negative, judging, or fearful in some way.

Remember that you have been training in "wild mind" for a long time. These practices will allow the mind to settle and the clouds of thought to dissipate. It doesn't have to happen all at once—but it *will* happen if you remain present and continue noticing what arises, with gentle curiosity and unconditional acceptance.

You have an unlikely ally in this process—your own emotions. We will turn to the arena of emotion in the next chapter, and see how feelings can serve as a guide to let us know when we have been taken off course by our thought patterns.

We will explore the natural role of emotions, both pleasant and unpleasant, and learn how to have a full experience of a feeling so that its effects are short-lived. When the winds of emotion are strong and damaging, as is inevitable, you need a way to hold yourself steady. You will learn how to keep yourself from being tossed about by emotional storms, minimizing the harm they can cause.

9

Step 5: Turn Toward the Feeling

How to Remain Steady Even in Tough Times

If there is one single emotion at the core of the human experience, it is fear.

—EDWARD HALLOWELL

Key Points

- Emotions are thoughts residing in the body. They cause distress only when they become stagnant or overwhelmingly strong.
- Emotions are meant to flow through the body like a stream or rise and fall like a wave. Paying attention to their physical sensations allows them to flow more freely.
- If we are caught unaware by a strong negative feeling, it can quickly engage our personal "story" and increase the momentum of the emotion.
- Greater awareness allows for new responses to unpleasant emotions that can break the habitual patterns of emotional reactivity.

AS WE progress in the Resilience Training Program, we build upon the psychology of mindfulness to become more skilled at dealing with difficult situations, moods, and mental states—the kind that can trigger a more serious episode of anxiety. We seek to create a sense of safety and stillness so that we can open more fully to difficult experiences and not let ourselves be controlled by them.

Emotionally charged situations tend to trigger our preferred form of *emotional reactivity*. For some of us, it may mean shutting down to avoid feelings. Others speed up so much that stress overrides other feelings—another form of avoidance. Still others substitute one painful feeling, such as anxiety or disconnection, for another, such as loss or anger.

Each of us has our own patterned reaction, and if we took the time to notice, we would realize that it leads nowhere. It takes us on the same circular path that we have traveled over and over again without resolution.

This pattern can be modified through mindfulness practice, which empowers us to:

- Become aware of our habitual modes of thought. This awareness allows us to change the pattern.
- Recognize the connection between thoughts and emotions.
- Experience emotions as fleeting events that can be felt and released.
- Learn to turn toward difficult emotions with courage and equanimity.

When you become mindful of your emotions, the circular pathway begun by a negative feeling can become a fresh experience. Instead of unconsciously going in circles, you will see that the path includes a series of choice points, and in any given moment you may choose to go somewhere new, to do something different. In this way, you can gain a greater sense of control over your own emotional reactions. You can reclaim your emotional freedom.

Becoming Emotionally Skilled

At our initial visit, Ken started taking several calming supplements and began a mindfulness practice. When he returned for his follow-up appointment, he was clearly feeling better. "I feel quiet for the first time in my life," Ken said. However, he found that having a calm mind was unfamiliar and a little confusing: "It feels so strange. I don't really know what to do with it."

Ken had a history of trauma at a younger age. He had done years of therapy, and it helped him make sense of his life and come to a feeling of peace with his past. But until now nothing had quieted the constant noise in his head—not even the numerous medications he had tried.

Ken experienced dramatic improvement from natural therapies— the same ones described in chapter 5. With a calmer mind he was able to do mindfulness practices—such as awareness of breathing and ob- serving his thoughts—more easily than ever before. He had tried them in the past, but had been so mentally restless that it had felt pointless to him to continue.

But now he felt different, and while it was a huge relief, it was also troubling him. "With this stillness, I can feel things for the first time. I had no idea that I even *had* emotions. Frankly, I don't know what to do with them."

Ken's experience is not unusual. I've met very few people—either in the consulting office or in the rest of life—who are skilled with their emotions. Most of us are able to enjoy good feelings, but we are often dismayed when they end. And dealing well with difficult and unpleas- ant emotions is a challenge that few have mastered.

Feelings Begin in the Mind

Thoughts tend, then, to awaken their most recent as well as their most habitual associates.

—WILLIAM JAMES

Ken went on to describe a recent work encounter—one that had triggered a strong emotional reaction. He had returned to work after his vacation to find that a number of things had piled up in his absence. He had sensed for some time now that there was tension between him and his boss. When he encountered his boss for the first time after his return, Ken got a terse comment about needing to "get on top of things" quickly, as there were deadlines looming. He had expected something along the lines of "Welcome back. How was your vacation?" Instead, he felt dismissed, unappreciated—and quite insecure.

"It was weird—I could actually *feel* it. In the past, I would have just gotten more revved up, more stressed. I would have had no clue what I was feeling emotionally." Now Ken was aware that he felt bad. But he still had no idea what the feelings were or what to do with them.

Ken was understandably dismayed by his experience. Like most of us, he didn't *want* to feel bad. But his newfound awareness also gave him the opening he needed to reclaim his emotional life. When painful emotions arise unconsciously and automatically, we are captive to them—as Ken had been. But by practicing awareness and bringing mindfulness to this process, we can release the hold that such emotions have on us.

Painful emotions, including sadness, anger, or fear, are felt in the body—but the *source* of these feelings is the mind. Once a painful feeling takes hold, it is common to generate more negative thoughts around it. When we feel bad, the mind automatically kicks into gear and looks for reasons: *Why do I feel so bad?* And because the mind is so good at finding what's wrong, it can easily come up with something. Usually the thoughts are self-critical, harsh, and judging. Sometimes the mind creates distorted beliefs, like *I've always been this way. I'll always be this way. Other people don't have this problem—it's just me.* Such thoughts make us feel even worse.

Since these feeling are generated by the mind, there is also a straightforward way out of this dilemma—*recognizing thoughts as thoughts.* Practicing awareness of thinking, as described in the last chapter, is one of the best ways to free yourself from unpleasant emotions. If you are feeling neutral one moment and the next moment you feel out of sorts in some way, you know that you are caught up in your thinking mind. The negative feeling is a cue to observe your thoughts.

Let's return to Ken's example. If his awareness had been strong in the moment that his boss made the comment, he would have sensed the arising of emotions in his body. That could have reminded him to look at his thoughts and see how they led to his emotional reaction. Rather than beating himself up about it, he could simply say to himself, *Ah, I'm just thinking . . . nothing more.* He would still feel bad for a bit, but the feelings would have stopped growing and then could have quickly receded.

It all happens so fast that it is difficult to do this in real time, particularly since our awareness tends to be clouded by uncomfortable feelings. But you can use unpleasant feelings as a guide, telling you that there is something awry with your thoughts. If you turn on the light of awareness at this early stage, a minor twinge of emotion remains just that. Unpleasant emotions are like waves that rise, fall, and leave your consciousness—if you let them.

Cultivating Emotional Wisdom

This being human is a guest-house.
Every morning a new arrival.
Welcome and entertain them all!
Even if they're a crowd of sorrows.

—RUMI

It is common in our culture to believe that we should feel good at all times, even to see unpleasant feelings as a sign of failure. The psychology of mindfulness offers a more balanced view of what we usually label as "negative" emotions.

- Unpleasant feelings are a natural, normal part of being human.
- They arise seemingly out of nowhere, often unexpectedly. Each is to be welcomed, even treated as an honored guest.
- Those feelings that we consider bad or unpleasant are just as important as those that feel good.
- Some painful feelings (e.g., grief) may perform a vital function, such as clearing us out so that something else can come in.
- Other feelings (e.g., fear) can guide us if we attend to them. They can serve as messengers, key sources of information that we ought to heed.
- Normal emotions, like guests, are meant to stay only a while. After being entertained or attended to, they will leave.

We need *all* of the emotions, those that feel good as well as those that don't feel good. They can guide us, letting us know when we are being harmed by others (or ourselves), when we need to change a situation that we are in, or when there is some misperception or other error in our thinking. Emotions can also empty us out when they are fully felt, clearing the way for a new and fresh experience as soon as a different feeling arises.

It is normal and healthy to have a full range of emotions—but that doesn't mean that they have to last. You can attend to your emotions, receive whatever they have to offer, and then allow them to leave. You do this by turning toward the feeling.

Having a Complete Experience of the Emotion

Ken wasn't sure he liked the idea of really experiencing his emotions. "I've been trying for years to get some emotional relief. Now I've got it—why would I want to feel bad again? Shouldn't I be able to stop myself from having bad feelings?"

I could understand why this seemed frightening to Ken. After all, he had gone through times where his emotions had knocked him off his feet. But these were not overwhelming feelings. What Ken described were just uncomfortable but normal emotions. They could lead to something worse if not attended to. But if Ken turned toward them right away, these mildly unpleasant feelings would quickly pass, leaving him unharmed.

You can't prevent feelings from arising any more than you can stop yourself from having thoughts. But you can develop a skillful way of responding to them. You can turn your awareness toward the emotion, not so as to figure out what is going on or what to do about it, but just to *have a complete experience of the emotions themselves*. This allows the feelings to have their moment of life but to move through you without getting stuck. In this way, even negative emotions can flow naturally and effortlessly.

They can even leave you feeling cleansed. Healthy grieving is a good example of this. With grief, we intuitively know that it needs to be felt, in all its fullness, if we are to be healed again. With practice, we can apply this full awareness to all of the emotions.

Ken was not ready to do this in the heat of the moment, when his feelings first arose during the encounter with his boss. Such awareness requires more practice, and he can cultivate this ability. But he got much of the same benefit by sitting with these feelings *after* the incident had occurred. The emotions may still be on the surface or they may have gone underground, but so long as they are still present in us, the feelings will need to be acknowledged, felt, and released.

Mindfulness teacher Shinzen Young describes three basic stages in attending to emotions: "We start by making the experience tangible, then noticing how it changes, and finally yielding to that change. That is a complete experience of emotion."[1]

Embodiment: Making the Feeling Tangible

"What I mean by turning toward the emotion," I explained to Ken, "is to place your awareness directly on the feeling—just as you do when you place your awareness on your breath. Begin by turning your attention toward your body, where the feeling arises.

"At first, it may seem like a confused jumble—you just know that you feel uncomfortable, but can't distinguish anything more. But if you stay with it, you will begin to notice *where* in the body you feel bad— usually somewhere between the throat and the groin, though it could be anywhere.

"Then you can start to distinguish between one feeling and another. What *particular* kind of uncomfortable feeling is it? Can you feel the difference between sadness, loss, disappointment, fear, anger, shame, and so on? What sort of pain do you feel—is it heavy, sharp, dull, soft, or something else?

"You can also notice the *strength* of the feeling. Is it intense, moderate, or mild? And does that intensity change as you watch it?"

Noticing in this way is fairly simple, and anyone can develop this skill. The ability to be aware of physical sensations is something we all have but usually don't practice. It is the same as being aware of the breath, sounds, or tastes. With just a little guidance and practice, you can quickly become adept at this.

Simply placing your attention on the feeling changes it, especially if you do so with pure awareness—that is, without letting the mind seize up in fear or judgment. It is a bit like being a scientist, interestedly observing a natural phenomenon but not being attached to it. *The very act of observing a process changes it.* This is particularly true when it is your own awareness observing your own inner experience.

Impermanence: Everything Changes, Including Emotions

One of the main principles of Buddhist teaching, *impermanence*, says that nothing stays the same—and that includes your emotions. That is hard to believe if you're in the midst of a bad mood that feels as if it is here to stay.

It is helpful to understand impermanence on an intellectual level, but much more useful is to actually experience it for yourself. In the guided meditation to follow, you can learn to do just that. Observing the emotion change, move, ebb, and flow makes it clear that even a bad feeling doesn't last.

The notion of fully experiencing painful feelings can be frightening to someone who has gone through a severe emotional disturbance such as an anxiety attack or a depressive episode. Remember that right now we are working with the *normal* emotions—not overwhelming feelings such as panic or despondency. That requires a different set of skills, which we will discuss later. But if you engage your awareness early in the process, with the first hint of insecurity, self-doubt, or nervous surveillance, the negative emotion may never grow into anything more ominous.

Yielding: Giving Way to the Flow

It is paradoxical that giving in to the emotion, rather than resisting it, can actually free you of it. Yielding does not mean giving up or submitting to an unwelcome emotion. It means letting the emotion flow, allowing it to rise and crest like a wave and then recede.

Confidence will come from experiencing for yourself that a so-called negative emotion, fully felt, can simply move on. Once it has been given your attention it can leave—its purpose has been served and you can release it. Then you are ready for the next moment, fresh and cleansed, aware and waiting for whatever experience your life brings you.

Mindfulness Practice: Awareness of Emotions

This is a meditation on feeling and fully experiencing the emotions. You will use many of the same skills that you learned with the mindfulness meditation in the last chapter, but will focus on emotional feelings instead of thoughts.

You will invite a feeling to arise and turn your awareness toward that feeling. Work with an unpleasant emotion, but not one that is too strong or difficult. You may need to engage your imagination and remember a recent emotional experience, unless there is a feeling right on the surface that you wish to work with.

There is no need to be frightened by these feelings. If something arises that seems too strong, you may choose to return your awareness to the breath. When you feel ready, you can invite some other, less intense feeling or memory to arise. You have complete freedom to do whatever you need with this meditation.

- Get into whatever position you wish, using a chair, cushion, or bench.
- Check your position to see if you need to shift it to be more comfortable.
- Begin with a few moments of awareness of breathing. Use the breath as your touchstone, returning to it when you realize that your mind has wandered off, and stay with the breath until you have regained your conscious awareness.
- Recall the image of your observing self, sitting by the banks of a river watching thoughts rise and fall. In this meditation, you will instead observe the rising and falling of emotions.
- Invite a difficult emotion to arise—one that has a negative charge for you but is not too strong. It may be a mild feeling of anger, a small sadness or loss, an annoyance, a fear of some sort. It might help to remember some difficult encounter or unpleasant situation that generated the feeling. You can play it back in your mind with as much detail as you can.
- As your mind generates thoughts and feelings about this situation, try to track the physical sensations that occur.

- What is the quality of the sensation? Does it feel hot, prickly, heavy, pressured, something else? How does anger differ from fear or from sadness?
- Where in the body does the feeling seem to settle? How does it move? Is it stuck or flowing? Just notice your experience without judging it.
- How strong is it? Observe how the strength changes, how the intensity goes up and down. What seems to affect the strength of the feeling?

- Notice how emotion rises and falls like a wave. Similar to the breath, there is expansion and contraction. Try to ride the wave, neither suppressing it nor fanning it with your thoughts. Just sit with it as it rises and falls.

- If thoughts begin to take you out of the experience of the emotion, just try to notice that, and return your awareness to your body and physical sensations.

- Notice all the ways that the emotion is changing—the location, the flow, the intensity—nothing stays the same.

- As best you can, give yourself over fully to the emotion. Yield to it; allow it to move and flow, to build momentum, reach a crest, and then recede.

- If you have such an experience of the emotion, notice how you feel after it has receded. How has your body changed after the emotion has left?

- If you have not felt as though you've had a complete experience of the emotion, know that you may return to it and work it through at your own pace.

- Whatever your experience has been, that is okay. Again, there is no success or failure. You are simply bringing awareness to your inner experience, with kindness and tenderness toward yourself.

Surviving Emotional Storms

Let everything happen to you: beauty and terror. Just keep going. No feeling is final.

—RAINER MARIA RILKE

Until now, we have been considering the normal range of human emotions. But there are other emotions that are far too strong to be considered normal waves—they are more like tidal waves, emotional tsunamis. Everyone has them—those times in life when the intensity of an emotion knocks us off our feet, and we wonder if we can get back up.

How can you remain steady until the wave has passed, minimize its damage, and regain your bearings? How is it possible to lessen the harmful energy in these storms?

Elena was about fifty years old when she began looking for new ways to deal with her lifelong anxiety, which included panic attacks and occasional depression. She was on several medications, which did little to keep her anxiety at bay.

She had never heard of mindfulness and had not yet begun the Resilience Training Program when she related the following experience. It illustrates several of the choice points where one could apply mindfulness skills to slow the oncoming wave of an emotional tsunami.

Elena had been feeling well until the day before our appointment. But that afternoon—"in just thirty minutes!" she exclaimed—her mood turned from fine to frantic.

Elena grew up in another country and did not speak English well. She had found it hard to make friends in her new home and she felt isolated. That afternoon, she and her husband went for a short walk around their neighborhood. They stopped at the home of a woman from

Elena's own country whom she considered a friend. There she found another neighbor woman with her friend, and the two were having tea.

Immediately Elena felt hurt because she hadn't been invited. She felt left out and vaguely threatened by this. Then she became angry and confronted her friend, which led to an argument between them. Later, as she and her husband walked home, she yelled at him because he didn't support her view of what had just occurred.

Many of us can relate to this story and understand why Elena felt hurt and left out. But look at the result—her mood went from good to horrible in just a few moments. Had anything actually changed in her life? Her husband was the same person he had been before. Her friends and neighbors were no different. She was no worse off, on the surface, than she had been a half hour earlier.

What had changed was her mind. Whereas it had been relatively peaceful, now it was agitated and filled with thoughts of not being liked, not having friends, never being able to fit in to this culture— and having an unsupportive husband as well.

Elena felt helpless, and in a sense she was. Because the mind is so powerful, if it is allowed to run rampant like this, then we are truly helpless in the face of it.

Breaking the Cycle of Painful Emotions

It is inevitable that we will experience emotions such as anger, fear, sadness, hurt, frustration, embarrassment, shame, guilt, and impatience. And they will occasionally be strong, even overpowering. If we lose our bearings during such a time, the suffering mind creates a state of emotional confusion. Then we are not only unable to find a way out of the situation but also at risk of making it worse. Unwise actions, such as Elena confronting her friend or getting angry with her husband, can turn an unpleasant situation into a long-term problem.

The way that the mind reacts to such painful emotions has a great deal to do with our resilience. When the mind is highly reactive, as it was for Elena in the moment described, it can easily trigger old habits of thinking. And this can quickly cascade into unhealthy beliefs such as *I am unworthy and unlovable*. This emotional reactivity is one of the primary causes of relapse of anxiety or depression.

Having the courage to remain present in the face of such powerful emotions gives you leverage over them. There are several points along the way where mindful awareness can rob the wave of its momentum. Even if you have been entirely swept away, it is never too late to bring in mindfulness and reduce your suffering.

Attachment to Experience

There are six sources of experience: the five sense perceptions of sight, smell, hearing, touch, and taste, and then the mind, which makes some kind of evaluation of these experiences. The sense perceptions are always active, and the mind is busy judging each perception in one of three ways: as pleasant, unpleasant, or neutral. That is just part of the mind's job, and that in itself is not a problem.

The problem arises when the mind becomes attached to experience, wanting things to be a certain way and feeling unhappy when they aren't. So when the experience is pleasant, we want more of it. This is called *grasping*. When it is labeled as unpleasant, we want to push it away. This is known as *aversion*. And sometimes, when the mind's label is neutral, the reaction is to become unconscious. This is sometimes called *delusion*, but a more descriptive term might be *mindlessness*.

In Elena's example, she reacted mainly with aversion—she did not want things to be as they appeared, and her mind created feelings of hurt, anger, and resentment. She was also grasping—wanting so badly to be included that she felt threatened by being left out. And she acted mindlessly when she allowed herself to speak angrily to others.

With mindfulness, the intention is to leave it at "pleasant," "unpleasant," or "neutral" so that attachment does not grow into a full-blown emotional storm as it did for Elena. You can simply consider something to be pleasant without feeling threatened if you don't have it; to be unpleasant instead of becoming critical or resentful; or as neutral instead of becoming bored or restless.

A wiser reaction to a stressful experience is known as *non-attachment*. That term does not mean that we are passive or indifferent. But it does mean that we are able to see and accept things as they are, while still being free to respond to them consciously if need be. This allows for greater emotional steadiness, preventing us from getting swept away by an emotional reaction.

Interrupting the Momentum: Finding Moments of Choice in a Storm

Three little fish are staring at a hook dangling before them. One of them is saying: "Remember—the secret is non-attachment."

—*NEW YORKER* CARTOON

Buddhist teacher Pema Chodron describes emotional reactivity as "getting hooked." We can't always stop ourselves from taking the bait, but we can still train ourselves to "interrupt the momentum, the escalation of suffering."[2] This involves bringing awareness into several different points during the rise of an emotional storm so that we can consciously choose to disrupt its escalation.

Let's examine Elena's situation further, to consider where you could apply mindfulness in your own similar cycles and slow the momentum of the storm.

The Initial Surge of Emotion

Elena's mood was neutral until the moment she realized that her friend was with someone else. Then an emotion began to arise, as automatically as a thought. At first there was just a vague sense of feeling bad. If she paid attention, she would notice an inner tightening—a sign that she is resisting her experience. If she could keep herself focused on this initial reaction, turning her attention inward, it might stay right where it is and eventually dissipate. At least it might not grow any stronger.

This first stage is the most subtle and difficult, but it is the most powerful in terms of reducing harm. The skill is simply to notice that you are tightening or pulling away, that this is going beyond "pleasant," "unpleasant," or "neutral." You cannot stop this first upwelling of emotion, because it arises automatically, seemingly out of nowhere. As soon as you notice the arising of feeling, let it signal you to remain still, to just stay right with your experience before things escalate further.

The Entering of Thought

Elena began to think: *She invited this neighbor, but not me. I have invited her to my place for tea. Why am I left out?* Once a painful emotion has taken hold, the mind kicks into gear and further negative thoughts arise. If allowed, this just adds fuel to the fire. If she were able to observe her thoughts, she could remind herself: *These are only thoughts.* That takes the mind out of gear so it stops escalating the emotion.

At this second level you are becoming caught up by the emotion. But the storm is still brewing and the emotions haven't yet reached full strength. Perhaps there is a slight pain in the heart or tensing in the throat, a feeling of being irritated or mildly upset. If it hasn't yet been fueled by the thinking mind, you could keep it right there by letting the thoughts go and coming back to pure awareness of the experience. Feel whatever you are feeling and accept it as it is.

Getting Caught Up in Your Story Line

Elena unconsciously began to build a case for why she felt so bad. *I never get asked to tea. I have no friends here. I'm unlikable. I'm unworthy.* When she feels threatened or hurt, old story lines come in: *These things always happen to me. There is something wrong with me.* This sense of unworthiness or being deeply flawed quickly accelerates the buildup of the mood. If Elena could recognize that her story has become engaged, she could still reduce its harm. By returning her awareness to the actual inner experience of the moment, she could feel all that is happening without judgment or fear.

When you become swept away by an emotion in this way, it means that your personal story line is getting triggered. At this point, you can still recognize that you are thinking or feeling hurt. You can see that you are getting caught up in your story. Try to identify with the observer within you—the part of you that is not caught up in all the drama. Seeing what is going on and identifying it, you can still calm the fires of the negative emotion. The best thing you can do is to stay with your moment-to-moment experience.

Speaking or Acting

Elena acted out of her emotion, blaming her friend and becoming angry with her husband. This damaged her relationships, creating further isolation. If the surge of emotion becomes too strong, it is hard to resist *doing* something. Once she speaks or acts, she easily causes further harm to herself and others. If possible, Elena could remind herself to be still. When firmly in the grip of an unhealthy mood, it is usually best to do nothing until you can regain your bearings.

At this stage, you are just about to talk or act. The emotion and the story that goes with it have taken over your mind and body and yell at you: *Don't just sit there—do something!* Instead, when the urge arises in your mind, do not act and do not speak. Remain still. As the Buddhists say, don't just do something—sit there! This is not the same as repression or denial, because you are doing this consciously and intentionally. It takes great courage to even attempt to interrupt the wave at this point. But with motivation and practice, you can do it, and prevent further injury to yourself or others.

After the Fact

Even after going through all the above stages, Elena could go back over it in her mind to see what had happened and where things could have gone differently.

Even after being overtaken by a toxic mood, even if you've acted or spoken and the damage has been done, it is still not too late to apply mindfulness. For most of us, working after the fact is the easiest place to start with this practice. Once you are removed from the situation, you can sit down and replay the experience—not to restimulate the painful feelings, but just to get in touch with that initial surge of emotion. Then you can mentally go through the same experience but imagine changing each of the stages by remaining calm and steady and not acting it out. Rehearsing in this way helps build the skills that you can eventually use in real time.

Remaining Present Is a Practice

All of us have repetitive emotional patterns that we cycle through unconsciously. It takes several repetitions to become aware that there even *is* a pattern. Be easy on yourself for letting this chain reaction sweep you along with its momentum—it can't be stopped entirely. The key is to acknowledge when you're being swept away, refrain from adding fuel to the fire, and remain still until a wise action becomes clear.

Mindfulness helps you stand your ground in the face of emotional storms. You build a foundation of inner strength that can keep you from being helplessly swept away by a painful mood. By practicing in this way, future storms will pack less of a punch.

Meanwhile, choosing awareness during *any* stage of an emotional storm will disrupt its pattern and deplete its energy. Do something different from the usual reactions, something fresh. Open to the painful experience, and in the next moment you may find that you are free of it. The practice is simply coming back to the present moment over and over again, so that it becomes a way of life.

Mindfulness Practice: Non-Attachment to Emotion

This is a meditation on remaining steady in an emotional storm. You will invite yourself to work with a challenging emotion. Choose a painful experience from which you have a safe distance.

There is no need to be frightened by these memories. If something arises that feels too strong, you may choose to return your awareness to the breath. When you feel ready, you may invite some gentler feeling or memory to arise. You have complete freedom to do what you need with this meditation.

Remember that you do have an anchor in the storm: you can ground yourself in your own body and your moment-to-moment experience. When you feel a welling up of a painful emotion, you can use awareness of breathing or any other physical sensation to ground you in the moment.

- Get into whatever position you wish, using a chair, cushion, or bench.
- Sit comfortably, back upright but not rigid. Check your position and see if you need to shift it to be more comfortable or more upright and alert.
- Begin with a few moments of grounding yourself. Notice the weight of your body; feel it being supported by the chair, bench, or cushion. Experience yourself being held, supported from below. You may notice how your hands are resting on your lap or the armrests of your chair. Feel the gentle pressure of it. Notice the feeling of warmth. Sense the texture of the fabric of your clothing.
- You may wish to expand your awareness to include the feel of the air around you. Sense its warmth or coolness, the slight movement of air in the room.
- Listen for any sounds around you or from within—the movement of air, breathing, coughing, shuffling, traffic noises from outside. Anything that enters your awareness can bring you into the moment.
- You may also turn your awareness to the breath and use that as your anchor. Experience the rising and falling of the breath.

- You can return to any of these experiences if you need to ground yourself again. Just tune in to the body, to a physical sensation, knowing that you can return to the present moment at any time.

- Now invite a memory to arise of a time when you experienced a strong or painful emotion—a memory that still feels charged but not overwhelming.

- If the feelings begin to get too strong, just return your awareness to some part of your physical experience in the present moment until you feel ready to return to the memory.

- We'll try to break it down into stages, even though it may have happened so fast. Start at the beginning of the memory—even before the mood arose, if you can. Who were you with, what were you doing, what were you wearing? Were there any sounds or smells that you recall? Bring it back in as much detail as you can.

- See if you can notice the very first welling up of emotion in you. It may be just a slight tightening up inside, or a desire to pull away from your experience. What is the feeling? You can put a label on it if that's helpful. Is it anger? Sadness? Fear? Insecurity? Shame? Something else? How does it affect you? Where is it in your body? How does it move?

- See yourself as fully present in this moment, without fear of the emotion. As you notice the feeling arise, know that you can remain still. See yourself holding steady in the face of the feeling, not letting it shake you off your moorings, until the feeling dissipates.

- Now let yourself imagine that the storm keeps growing. Your mind reacts automatically and you begin thinking, and that makes the emotion stronger. See yourself remaining still, not caught up in the thoughts or believing them, but able to sit and watch the process unfold, again without fear. You are able to observe in stillness, see the thoughts arise, not get carried away with them, and let them go.

- You can safely imagine that the emotional storm continues to grow and that you begin getting caught up in your own story, the same one you've entertained over and over again—as we all do. What are the themes? The hurts? The fears? Let them arise now, so that you can look at them and learn to take yourself out of the drama. To do this, try to identify with the observer in you. Try to see thought as just thought, feeling hurt as feeling hurt, feeling scared as feeling scared. When you see clearly what is going on, without being hard on yourself, you take the energy out of the emotion.

- Now imagine that this experience continues to unfold. Imagine that the feelings have strengthened so much that you are about to do or say something. It arises as an impulse, but you have enough presence to notice it before you do it. See yourself holding this impulse, reminding yourself to remain still. *Do nothing, just sit with this for now. I can act later, when my mind has cleared.*

- And even if you did act or speak, remember that it is never too late to become more aware, more mindful, more present. As soon as possible, find a time like this for a quiet reworking of the experience.

- Accept the experience just as it is. Things don't have to be any certain way. Be kind to yourself and grateful for this time, however it has been.

Step 6: Cultivate a Good Heart

How Self-Acceptance Leads to Greater Peace

Love is the great work
Though every heart is first an apprentice.

—HAFIZ

Key Points
- Emotional suffering is kept alive by the false belief that we are somehow flawed or inadequate.
- Genuine self-acceptance creates an inner sense of safety and sufficiency, the conditions for lasting resilience.
- Holding compassion for others is transformative, as it replaces an unhealthy focus on the self.
- Expressing kindness is healing both to the one who gives and the one who receives.

THIS CHAPTER marks a turning point in the practice of the psychology of mindfulness. Until now we have focused upon the role of the mind in creating unnecessary suffering. We have learned to observe thoughts and feelings without becoming triggered by them. We have practiced letting emotions flow through us when we are able and holding our ground when they are overpowering. The intention behind those practices is to become more skillful with our thoughts and feelings so that they cause us less harm.

Now we shift our attention beyond the relief of suffering. True health is more than the absence of illness. True resilience means more than *not* being stressed, anxious, or depressed. It is also possible to enlarge ourselves, to become more than we are at this moment or have been in the past. We can grow beyond recovery to being more fully alive, more fully ourselves.

Everyone has the capacity to have a "good heart"—one that is open, engaged, and loving. It is a very strong antidote to stress. It allows us to be at peace, to feel safe and secure, to know deep within that all will be well. Such positive inner states can be cultivated intentionally.

Having a good heart is completely natural, yet it takes practice. The process begins by holding the intention to become an open, loving person. It evolves through inner practices such as the meditations described in this chapter. We will focus on three specific practices that support the creation of a loving, open heart: self-acceptance, loving-kindness, and compassion.

We must begin with ourselves, but that is not where this transformation ends. A good heart does not keep to itself. It reveals itself by doing acts of kindness—both for ourselves and for others. A compassionate heart cannot help but *act*.

The Threat from Within

Leslie wasn't aware that she had a problem with anxiety. She went to her doctor complaining of tightness in her throat that she feared was a sign of some serious physical ailment. After a few tests were negative, the doctor suggested that it was anxiety that was causing her symptoms. They tried a couple of medications that only seemed to make things worse, and then she was referred to a therapist.

On the surface, everything in Leslie's life seemed fine. She was well educated and happily married, had successfully raised three children, and had a good network of supportive friends. She had never before felt a need to seek psychological help, and she didn't understand what could be causing anxiety—if in fact that's what it was.

With her therapist's help, Leslie began to realize that fear had actually ruled her life since childhood. Leslie had been raised in a tense home environment. She described her parents and even her siblings as being harshly critical of her. She could not recall ever being praised or told that her accomplishments were good enough. Instead, others were always finding fault with her.

From the perspective of adulthood, it makes little difference whether her family was actually critical of her or she just perceived them to be that way. Either way, those were the beliefs that she held about herself. Feeling that she never quite measured up to others' expectations, she had learned to carry those expectations within herself.

It was clear that Leslie was unhappy with herself, despite her outwardly good life. She described herself as a "shy and nervous person." Because she judged these qualities negatively, they provided further proof in her mind that something was fundamentally wrong with her. No matter how successful she was or how many good things she had in her life, she *felt* inadequate.

"Imagine that you could actually feel okay with yourself just as you are—with your body, your mind, your job, your relationships, your behaviors, and your shyness and nervousness, too. Would you still be unhappy?" I asked Leslie.

"It's possible, but there wouldn't be much energy behind it. I don't think it would last so long," she replied.

What kept Leslie's fear and discontent alive was not rooted in truth. Both were fed by her own unquestioned belief that, at a very deep level, she was not okay. With such beliefs, how *could* she feel secure in the world?

There are many like Leslie, who perceive the outside world as threatening and unsafe. Sometimes it is. Yet external threats come and go, while the feelings of being unsafe and inadequate can live on.

The ongoing source of threat is really in our own mind, nurtured by the persistent idea that we are flawed and not adequate to the tasks before us. The central fear around which our lives revolve is *I am not all right*. This is frequently accompanied by two supporting beliefs: *Whatever is wrong with me must be fixed* and *It cannot be fixed; this condition will be with me always*. There is a sense of needing help, but being beyond help. That can feel hopeless.

Buddhist teacher and psychologist Tara Brach refers to the persistent sense of shame and self-rejection as "the trance of unworthiness."[1] Over years of conditioning, heightened by struggles with stress and anxiety, we become possessed by a sense of deep inadequacy, losing touch with the basic goodness that is our birthright. This "trance" brings with it a high degree of self-consciousness (even self-preoccupation) and interferes with making connections with others and developing a sense of belonging.

Yet it is possible that the feeling of not being good enough can open the door to healing. It lets you know that something *is* wrong— not that something is wrong with *you*, but rather with the way you *hold* yourself. If you can see this as a belief that does not serve you, and nothing more than a belief, then you can move in the direction of healing. You can learn to hold yourself differently.

The Strategy of Self-Improvement

All of you are perfect just as you are—and you could use a little improvement.

—SHUNRYU SUZUKI-ROSHI

Since it creates such internal distress to feel so bad about ourselves, we try various unskillful strategies to relieve ourselves of this discomfort. Some of these strategies are supported by society, such as being overly busy or perfectionistic. Others are clearly self-destructive, such as the addictions.

For millions in the West, the strategy we choose is self-improvement. There is a huge industry that promotes the notion that we are flawed and to be happy must fix ourselves through the latest pill, makeover, or self-help technique. If it is happiness that we seek, we believe that we must strive to become better than we are.

We are all imperfect. What matters most is not how deficient we are but how we relate to our deficiencies. If they create a sense of inadequacy, low self-worth, or shame, then they will almost certainly prolong emotional suffering. Yet fixing ourselves is not the answer. Self-improvement is a never-ending task that leads to a kind of inner imprisonment.

This is not to say that there is no role for good self-care. Much of what we do in the Resilience Training Program involves intelligently applying healthy self-care measures. But that can be done without the added notion *There is something wrong with me and I need to find it and fix it.*

This is the paradox we can choose to embrace. It is possible to accept yourself completely as you are and still work at becoming more healthy, peaceful, and kindhearted. You can make the inner shift from *I need to fix myself* to *I accept myself fully—now how can I feel better?* Acceptance is the key. It gives you the opening to make this shift.

Acceptance is almost magical in its power to release inner tension, let go of inner conflicts, and transform the way you hold yourself.

Seeing What Is: The Doorway to Self-Acceptance

Leslie had lived with unnecessary anxiety for decades because she was in denial of it. She wasn't even aware of its presence. Denial was her default mechanism, the strategy that automatically came into play when she reacted unconsciously to distress. Each of us has our own pattern of unconscious reactivity, usually some combination of the three "unskillful means" discussed in the last chapter: grasping, aversion, and mindlessness.

It is important to remember that all of us use these strategies for the same reason—because we are not conscious that we do so. Without sufficient awareness, we go to our default mechanism, whatever it is. It is the best we can do in the moment to protect ourselves.

The first step out of this emotional reactivity involves having the courage to see when we are lost in a strategy. This requires courage because it is never easy to "catch ourselves in the act," behaving in ways that we know are hurtful to us. We have to remember that we are doing so out of an innocent desire to feel better. We don't realize that we are actually harming ourselves, because we aren't conscious of it. We must learn to become aware of when a "strategy" has come into play.

We must pass through the doorway of self-acceptance before it is even possible to undertake a journey toward healing. It is the essential first step that makes the rest of the journey possible. Awareness allows us to see our emotional traps or blind spots, which then gives us the opportunity to do things differently. It is crucial, however, to do this without self-judgment. This is the critical difference between creating a true healing practice and just another attempt at self-improvement.

Holding Yourself with Kindness

Be kind to yourself, dear—to our innocent follies.
Forget any sounds or touch you knew that did not help you dance.
You will come to see that all evolves us.

—RUMI

Seeing the harm caused by your unconscious strategies places you on the road to freedom. Moving forward on that journey involves relating to yourself—including all your "innocent follies"—with warmth and kindness. It requires time, attention, care, patience, and forgiveness. You are *befriending* yourself.

After working with hundreds of people in this program, I am convinced of the crucial importance of genuine self-acceptance. For many, this runs counter to years of ingrained habits that have reinforced their idea of themselves as flawed. You can release these beliefs by holding yourself with tenderness, as described in the following meditation—and practicing it over and over again.

Mindfulness Practice: A Meditation on Self-Acceptance

This is a meditation on opening the heart and directing warmth and kindness toward yourself. This is the key to moving beyond insecurity.

- Get into whatever position you wish, using a chair, cushion, or bench. Sit comfortably, back upright but not rigid.
- Check your position and see if you need to shift it to be more comfortable or more upright and alert.
- There is no need to hold yourself rigidly. Just imagine that you are royalty, and hold yourself in a dignified way.

- Experience yourself being held, aware that you are supported from below.
- Focus upon several breaths, allowing your mind to settle.
- Experience the rising and falling, rising and falling of the breath. You can return to awareness of your breath at any time during the rest of this meditation, using breath as an anchor to bring you back to the present.
- Now bring your awareness to your heart center, the area in the middle of your chest, just below your breastbone. You can gently place your hand over this area if that helps direct your awareness.
- Notice whatever feeling arises in your heart, setting aside all judgment or need for your feelings to be different than they are. Just notice what is.
- Become aware of the degree of openness that you experience at this moment. When your heart is open, you may notice a sense of expansion, flowing, fullness, lightness, or warmth. If the heart is closed, it may feel tight, stagnant, empty, heavy, or cool. Try not to judge one condition as good and the other bad. Just notice and accept whatever is true for you now, and know that it will change.
- Now, keeping some awareness on the heart center, invite your imagination to come into play. Bring to mind a time in the recent past when you were moved by something— when your heart was opened. It may have been a book, a movie, a story you heard, a compliment or other kind word that was not expected, an act of kindness toward you or someone else—anything that made you feel compassionate, grateful, more open.
- Whatever it was, try to recall the experience now as

vividly as you can. See any other person involved. Where did it take place? Were there any smells, colors, or sounds?

- Experience, for as long as you like, the feeling that you had at the time—the feeling of being moved and opened.

- Invite your heart now to open further. Observe it. Experience the feeling that you have when it opens.

· If no specific image or memory came up for you, simply hold the intention to let the heart soften and open now, in this moment.

- Now, bring to mind an image of yourself, just as you are.

- With whatever degree of openness you have, fill your awareness with feelings of warmth toward yourself. Imagine that you are holding yourself with kindness.

- You may turn toward some area of difficulty that you have, something you don't like or wish were different about yourself or your life. See that difficulty as vividly as you can.

- In your own way, say, "Ah, yes . . . this." Allow it to be as it is.

- As you breathe, notice what you feel. If there is hurt, where does it reside? If there is tightening, where is that?

- Keep breathing, with an intention to allow things to be as they are.

- Notice where you feel vulnerable, and breathe into that place with an air of compassion for yourself.

- Let go of the image of difficulty, and sit for a few more moments with your awareness on your heart. Hold yourself with kindness and compassion.

- Accept this time however it has been, being grateful for whatever degree of kindness you have been able to direct toward yourself. It takes a tremendous amount of courage to be able to open our hearts to ourselves.

Loving-kindness Practice: The Heart of Mindfulness

There are two great aspects to the mindfulness tradition. In the previous two chapters we focused on the first of these, often known as *vipassana* or "insight meditation." It means to see things as they really are, and it teaches us to grow in awareness, pay attention to mental habits, and learn not to be controlled by them. We can see things more clearly when the mind is calm, when we shine the light of awareness onto that which was previously unseen, and when we free the mind from mental and emotional suffering. Then we can pay attention to what is. But this insight is not the whole answer as to how to align mind, heart, and spirit.

The second wing of mindfulness teaches a practice known as *metta* or "loving-kindness meditation." It complements the cultivation of a calm and resilient mind. *Metta* practice involves the intentional creation of a "good heart," one capable of kindness, generosity, and compassion. A heart that is open, a heart that can give and receive, a heart that is connected to yourself and to those around you—that is a heart that expects to be happy and secure.

In this practice, we are attempting to do more than be present, aware, and accepting. We are engaging the heart in the highest possible way. We are planting the heart with "good seeds," hoping to become more resilient and loving in the process. When things become difficult or painful in the future, as they will, what better companion than our own benevolent heart?

This is not a mental activity. It involves opening the heart, which may have closed itself off in response to feeling threatened. We don't do so on purpose, but when we feel threatened in some way, the heart closes. We draw ourselves, with our vulnerability, within. We shut ourselves off from the world around us. We do it innocently and unconsciously to protect ourselves. It may even be a wise and helpful response at the time.

Often we remain protected far longer than is helpful. Maybe the threat was so great, or it occurred so many times, that the heart remains closed off from others. Or perhaps it has been this way for so long that we have forgotten how to open up again. Whatever the cause, the heart must open again in order to fully live.

You cannot *force* it to open—it must be allowed to do so in its own time. There has to be a sense of safety. Some of that can come from outside you. You can pay attention to what sustains your heart. For example, notice how other people affect you, and choose to spend more time with those who are healthier for you. Learn what activities leave you feeling more peaceful and find more opportunities to do them. Experience the calming effect that nature has on you and connect with it in ways that you find most nourishing.

Still, opening occurs within. In mindfulness, the foundational practice for cultivating a good and open heart is the *loving-kindness meditation*. Also called a *friendliness* or *caring practice*, it involves placing your attention on the heart and then generating a feeling of love, kindness, or well-wishing. You start with yourself, then hold others in your awareness, and finally cultivate loving-kindness for all of creation.

It is important that this practice begins with yourself. You may have a hard time with that, thinking that it is selfish or self-centered to place yourself first, or to give this kind of consideration to yourself at all. Or it may feel awkward or inauthentic, perhaps because you don't feel you deserve these good things, or it is not truly what you believe about yourself.

This is a way of affirming the central role of self-acceptance in healing. It is not selfish or self-centered to do this. In fact, it is very practical. We must first care for ourselves, and open to ourselves, if we wish to be truly present and loving with others.

The Dhammapada, a text ascribed to Buddha, puts it this way: "Hatred cannot coexist with loving-kindness, and dissipates if supplanted with thoughts based on loving-kindness." Loving-kindness practice is offered as a form of self-therapy, meant to heal the troubled mind and heart, and to cultivate self-acceptance as well as love for others. It can have an immediate impact on mood, and can help free you from negative habitual thoughts, breaking the repetitive pattern of circular thinking about yourself. This is a powerful form of caring, and it develops the ability to give more of yourself to others.

Mindfulness Practice: Loving-kindness Meditation

The inner statements that you make during the meditation are not mantras or affirmations. They are more like blessings or prayers. It is pointing the mind in the direction that you want it to go. You make these statements without a sense of expectation that they will be true, or the fear that they won't. You try to make them just because it is what you wish for yourself and others. Even if you don't actually feel that way, it is good to set that intention in the heart over and over again. You need only to approach this meditation with whatever openness and willingness you have right now.

- Sit quietly in a comfortable position.
- Focus upon several breaths, allowing your mind to settle.
- Bring your awareness to the heart center.
- Notice whatever feeling is in the heart at this moment, and accept it just as it is.
- Keeping some part of your awareness on the heart, bring to mind an image of yourself, now or at some time in the past. Allow this image to become as clear as possible.
- In your mind's eye, invite this image of yourself to come closer to the heart. You can imagine that you are embracing this image of yourself.

- Holding yourself in this way, you may offer a blessing from your heart to this image: "May you be at peace. May you be free from suffering. May your heart be filled with loving-kindness. May your life be filled with joy."

- When you are ready, let this image dissolve in your awareness. Observe, for a moment, the feeling now in your heart. Then invite another image to arise, this time the image of a loved one, someone who is dear to you now or has been in the past. As before, invite this person into your open heart and give him or her your blessing.

- Continue in this way, progressing outward from your self. After a loved one, you may hold a mentor or teacher, someone who has had a positive role in your life. Next, someone more neutral, like a colleague or an acquaintance. Then, if you feel able, invite someone who has hurt you or about whom you have difficult or conflicted feelings. You may extend this to your neighborhood, the community in which you live, your country, and the world at large.

- Before ending, hold your awareness lightly in the heart center, just noticing what is there. If it feels open and warm, be grateful for that. If it does not, just accept that.

- Whatever this time has been like for you, accept it as fully as you can.

Stepping Out of "My Story": Awakening to Compassion

There is a Native American story that says there are two wolves dwelling in every human heart. One is driven by fear and seeks to meet its own needs, often at the expense of others. It is greedy, self-absorbed, and quick to anger. The other wolf is motivated by love and concern for others. It is generous, kind, and compassionate. The two are waging a battle inside us to see which will have the greatest influence over our nature. The one that grows strongest, the story says, is whichever one we feed the most.

Modern science tells a similar story. Sophisticated imaging tools including PET and fMRI scans give pictures of the brain in action. This has allowed scientists to determine what brain areas correspond to various functions. They have discovered that the prefrontal cortex helps set our emotional tone as well as the ability to be empathic to others.

The two sides of the prefrontal cortex create very different internal states. When the right prefrontal cortex is more active, we are caught up in ruminative, self-absorbed thinking. The corresponding emotions are highly negative, such as worry, sadness, and anger. When the left side becomes activated, the result is the opposite. The mind is calmer, the stress response is shut down, and emotions are positive—such as enthusiasm, happiness, and well-being.[2]

The "two wolves," it would seem, reside in the prefrontal cortex. The following studies show how strongly they are influenced by what we put into our minds. They reveal how important it is to take care about which one we feed the most.

The first study involved teenagers who played a violent video game. The researchers used a common, popular game—the kind that over 90 percent of teens play. In just thirty minutes of play, their fight-or-flight response became activated. Afterward they showed a lingering pattern of negative emotional arousal.[3] The teens' bodies reacted as though they were in an actual battle—their senses were heightened, hearts racing, muscles tensed. Though it is just a game, the brain can't tell the difference—it is "kill or be killed" so far as the brain is concerned. When the stress hormones are this high, the part of the brain involved with sound judgment and self-control is turned off. Concern for others fades into the background. The "good wolf" becomes quiet.

In a second series of studies, Buddhist monks were shown a photo of an infant with an obvious growth deformity on its skull. They were then given instructions to hold the infant with tender awareness, to fill their hearts and minds with nothing but compassion for this suffering being. As they did so, their brain metabolism was measured and showed a dramatic increase in activity of the left prefrontal cortex—the seat of compassion.

Later, participants with no meditation experience were given similar instructions. At first they showed very little capacity to activate the compassion center. But with simple meditation instructions and a small amount of practice, they became more adept at activating their left prefrontal cortex—not as dramatically as the monks who had practiced longer, but significant nonetheless.[4]

As the novice meditators turned their attention toward cultivating compassion for another, they also shut down the parts of their brain that cause stressful, unpleasant feelings. Instead, they created positive feelings such as emotional steadiness, openness, and empathy. Feeding the good wolf is possible for everyone. It simply requires attention and practice. Its positive effects are limitless.

Imagine for a moment the possibilities these studies create in your life. We have a choice as to how we feed our minds. What we choose has a great impact on our emotional state. We know intuitively that it feels better to be compassionate toward others than it does to be narrowly concerned with ourselves and our own survival. Now modern science confirms what meditation practitioners have known for centuries: working intentionally with our minds and hearts, we can become all that we wish to be.

Mindfulness Practice: A Meditation on Compassion

Being awake involves stepping out of the painful focus on ourselves and expanding our circle of care and compassion. Holding another with compassion transforms us.

- Get into whatever position you wish, using a chair, cushion, or bench. Sit comfortably, back upright but not rigid.
- Check your position and see if you need to shift it to be more comfortable or more upright and alert.
- Sit with awareness of your breath for a few moments.
- Next turn your attention toward your heart. Imagine that you are breathing in and out of your heart center.
- Notice whatever is in your heart. There is no need to change it. Accept your experience, and yourself, fully in this moment.
- Now bring to mind someone who you know is struggling in some way. Let the image of this person become very clear in your mind. Invite that image into your heart.
- If you know the nature of the person's suffering, hold that awareness without judgment. Remember that all of us struggle in similar ways.
- Try to fill your awareness with the wish that this person may be released from his or her suffering. Your mind may wander. Still, remain intent on being completely focused on the other.
- Sit for as long as you'd like with an openhearted awareness of the other person and a genuine desire to see his or her suffering relieved.
- Return your awareness to your own heart. Sit for a few moments with whatever is there, grateful for any opening you experienced.

Kindness:
The Universal Balm

Be kind. Everyone you meet is fighting a great battle.

—PHILO OF ALEXANDRIA

The Dalai Lama has been quoted as saying: "My religion is very simple. My religion is kindness." Indeed, life is so hard, how could we be anything *but* kind? That is poignantly true for those who have suffered for years with anxiety and other effects of stress. But shouldn't our focus be on receiving kindness if we are trying to heal? Why suggest acts of kindness as a means of recovering our own resilience?

Kindness is healing. It is helpful for those who receive it, of course. It is also healing to give it. This is one way of acting on the lessons from the neuroscientists. It feels good to get outside of our own small circle of concern and do something kind for another. It enlarges and enlivens us.

In the Resilience Training Program, we use a simple activity to build the capacity for kindness. I am grateful to my teaching colleague, Sandra Kacher, who designed the practice.

The Three Kindnesses Practice involves noticing when an act of kindness occurs. When you shift your attention toward it, you begin to realize that such acts are occurring all the time, all around us. It is easy to forget the ubiquity of kindness when there is so much violence, so much pettiness, so much meanness in the world. It is true that those exist. We are flooded with images, stories, and news reports to remind us of that. Yet the other, kinder side of life is just as real. It becomes more so as we turn our hearts toward it.

Mindfulness Practice: Three Kindnesses

This is a practice of witnessing the goodness of events as they unfold during your routine encounters. Set the intention to notice acts of kindness when they occur. When you do see an act of kindness, allow yourself to be struck by it. Write it down—this will help you to remember it, and also encourage the heightening of your awareness.

There are three different patterns to look for:

1. Someone acts kindly toward another person.
2. Someone acts kindly toward you.
3. You act kindly toward another.

Witnessing and taking note of such simple acts encourages them. Be especially attentive to your own actions toward others. You will find yourself being kind more readily, becoming more active in reaching out, and feeling better about yourself.

A good heart is something we all gain from. Turning our attention inward and seeing the goodness that is there—that is healing. Placing our awareness on the heart with the intention to open it—that is transforming. Holding others with compassion—that is liberating. Acting with kindness at every opportunity—that is joyful.

Doesn't everyone want these things? Isn't this what we long for, really? A good heart is open and full—and it wants to connect. We will turn toward this in the next chapter.

Step 7:
Create Deep Connections

How to Develop a Sense of Belonging in the Larger World

We can live without religion and meditation, but we cannot survive without human affection.

—THE DALAI LAMA

Key Points

- Resilience requires a genuine sense of belonging and engagement.
- When we are present, we can access deep calm at any moment, even difficult ones.
- If we listen to our inner voice, it will guide us toward the connection we seek.

IN THIS way, we are all alike: we want the same few things. Beyond what is needed to survive, we all want to feel connected and supported. We all want to have others show interest in us and appreciate us. We all want to feel part of things, to belong.

Being connected in this way is perhaps the most healing and life-giving of all the aspects of resilience. Without it, as the Dalai Lama said, we cannot survive. Or at least we cannot survive well.

In this chapter we will touch upon three lessons from the psychology of mindfulness that teach us about creating deep connections:

1. Replacing the idea of separation with an awareness of unity.
2. Becoming more fully present to one another through deep listening.
3. Becoming more fully present to oneself by attending to the inner voice.

Belonging to the World

The *Tao Te Ching* paints a picture of a healthy society, one that is "governed wisely," where belonging comes naturally: "People enjoy their food, take pleasure in being with their families, spend weekends in their gardens, delight in the doings of the neighborhood."[1]

On a recent Mother's Day I shared such an experience. I went with my family to a large city park to celebrate the occasion. It was a beautiful spring day, and the park was filled with groups of people enjoying themselves. They looked as if they had originated from all over the world. Many wore colorful ethnic dress and appeared to be there with extended families that included all the generations. Each gathering had bountiful food. Children were everywhere and the sounds of conversation and laughter filled the air.

Though we didn't know anyone else there, it was a joy just to walk around and soak it in, feeling part of this celebration of life. This felt like the kind of world we wish to live in—the shared world. In such an idyllic gathering, it is hard to imagine not feeling happy and at ease. There is something so peaceful and reassuring about belonging. We need it to feel whole.

Neuroscientist Lou Cozolino makes a similar point in his book *The Neuroscience of Human Relationships*. He draws a parallel between a single nerve cell and an individual person, neither of which can survive in isolation:

> The individual neuron or a single human brain does not exist in nature. Without stimulating interactions, people and neurons wither and die. In neurons this is called apoptosis; in humans it is called depression, grief, and suicide. From birth until death, each of us needs others who seek us out, show interest in discovering who we are, and help us feel healthy and safe . . . relationships are our natural habitat.[2]

I believe that there is a great truth in this statement, one that we are reminded of during crises, such as when a community undergoes a natural disaster such as a flood. At times like those, people feel connected, and their natural, spontaneous reaction is to reach out in love and support.

Several years ago, sociologists studied small, tight-knit, traditional cultures where mental health problems such as anxiety and depression were extremely rare. They were looking for the factors that protected these people from illnesses that are so common in the West. They concluded that it was their close connection with one another that spared them from the destructive effects of stress. If one member of the group suffered, they all did: "Your pain is my pain." They responded to others' loss or hurt by caring, helping, supporting, and connecting with one another. In fundamental ways, they were one.

Reflecting on life as it is nearing its end provides another lens for what really matters. When asked if they would change anything in their life, dying people respond with statements such as "I wish I'd loved better" or "I would have spent more time with those who were really important to me."

One cannot overemphasize the importance of deep connection. Without it, it is impossible to withstand the stresses that we all face. No matter how pristine your diet, how strong your exercise, how deep your meditation practice, you cannot do well alone. Yet when there is deep connection, people can survive great catastrophe and remain resilient. It is the most protective, the most important of the roots of resilience.

The Second Great Mistake

Why are you unhappy? Because nearly everything that you say and do is for your "self"—and there isn't one!

—CHINESE PROVERB

Rick didn't *want* to go it alone—he couldn't seem to help it. He loved people, wanted to be around them, wanted to be part of things. Yet he couldn't shake the feeling that he didn't quite fit in. It had followed him his entire life, as closely as his shadow.

Rick had felt this way as far back as he could remember, and he didn't understand it. He was friendly, easy to talk to, and a good listener. Others enjoyed his company, and he had many friends. Why, then, did he feel himself to be so separate?

His belief that he was outside the circle of belonging gave Rick a deep sense of unease. As I came to know him better, it became clear that this was the true source of his general anxiety and unhappiness.

In the psychology of mindfulness, this idea that we are separate, isolated beings is considered an illusion. It is the second great falsehood, the first being the belief that we are deeply flawed and unworthy. It is hard to recognize this belief as an illusion, though, because nearly everyone else in our culture believes it to be true, too. Our Western minds are steeped in the values of individuation and independence. We hold firm to the idea of the rugged individual. We go it alone.

Without intending to do so, Rick had incorporated the values of his family and society. He had bought into the notion that there are not enough good things for everyone, so you have to protect your own. Deep down he believed that there really *are* winners and losers, that if another was successful, that meant he was not. Without meaning to be, he was quietly competitive in almost every area of his life. Despite his own success, he couldn't help but feel envious of those who seemed happier or more at ease than he was. The result of this unconscious activity was that the belonging he craved was even further out of his reach.

Waking Up from the Illusion

Our bodies know they belong; it is our minds that make our lives so homeless.

—JOHN O'DONOHUE

Unaware of what was driving his behavior, Rick had tried many strategies to fill the void within. At times he felt inferior and assumed that he wasn't good enough to belong. Then he would strive to better himself to the point of perfectionism, trying to prove that he was worthy. Work was a good way to do this. He worked extremely hard and was a successful physician. This proved his value in his own mind and at the same time kept him so busy that he didn't have time to develop close relationships.

Sometimes he would set himself apart by trying to be better than others, to be special in some way. Feeling superior spared him from the pain of being left out, but its effects didn't last. Soon his uneasiness would seep back in, driving him to some other unconscious attempt to make things right.

Rick did not know how to be any different, in part because he was unaware of the root of the problem. He didn't realize that he was clinging to a small notion of "self" at the expense of what he really wanted, which was to belong to something larger than himself.

There are some clues that can tell us when we have become caught up in the belief of separateness. When we compare ourselves to others, favorably or unfavorably, we are caught up in this belief. We know we are caught by it when we feel competitive, when we grasp or hoard, when we feel inadequate, insufficient, or insecure. We are also caught when we feel superior, critical, or rejecting of others.

When we think in terms of *mine* and *yours*, or focus on the differences between *them* and *us*, we are caught in the illusion of separation. When we are fearful of the other who is different from us, when we fear that we won't get our due, when we hold ourselves apart from others or feel we don't belong, when we feel depressed because we are lonely and isolated—we are caught in this illusion.

As Rick continued with his mindfulness practice, he began to see the real source of his lifelong uneasiness and sense of isolation. It was not because he was unlikable or unworthy. Nor was he special or set apart in some way. He was essentially no different from those he set himself apart from.

He realized that he created his own separateness by his thoughts and beliefs. Seeing this, he began to challenge them. The source of his isolation was his mind, and it was there that he could begin to create the openness for belonging.

Your Happiness Is My Happiness

Ordinary happiness depends on happenstance. Joy is that extraordinary happiness that is independent of what happens to us. Good luck can make us happy, but it cannot give us lasting joy. The root of joy is gratefulness.

—BROTHER DAVID STEINDL-RAST

If we wish to create "extraordinary happiness," we don't want to rely upon chance. As Rick found out, what we most long for does not necessarily occur on its own. Our misguided attempts to find it can instead push it further away. We have to attend to our inner lives in order to break down the walls of separation and create a space for gratefulness. To create the conditions for lasting happiness, we must begin with the mind.

One of the ways we can cultivate these conditions is to do a meditation practice often referred to as "sympathetic joy." It involves bringing people to mind, as we did in the loving-kindness practice. In this case, we practice being happy for their happiness or good fortune. We share in their joy.

The Dalai Lama points out that this is very practical. Why rely just on your own good fortune to be happy? If there are six billion people in the world and you can be happy for their good fortune, then you have just increased your chances of being happy by six billion times!

A practice like this counters the tendency to encircle our individual lives with a protective fence of self-concern. The capacity to experience the joy of another as if it were our own opens us to an unending supply of joy—the kind of happiness and satisfaction that do not depend upon what happens to us. It also takes us off the hook, since we no longer need to fix ourselves or be special in any way. We can replace envy and competition with generosity and abundance. We can join the circle.

Mindfulness Practice: A Meditation on Shared Joy

The belief in a separate self is one of the strongest obstacles to connection and belonging. Generosity is a potent antidote to this belief and the grasping that accompanies it. The conditions for generosity are created within by taking joy in the success or good fortune of others.

- Get into whatever position you wish, using a chair, cushion, or bench. Sit comfortably, back upright but not rigid.
- Check your position and see if you need to shift it to be more comfortable.
- Begin with a few moments of awareness of the breath, and use that to allow the mind to settle. You may return to the breath as your anchor as you continue.
- Bring your awareness to the heart center.
- Notice whatever feeling is in the heart at this moment, and accept it just as it is.
- Now bring to mind someone close to you who seems really happy or successful. Try to get as clear an image as you can. See the look of happiness or content on that person's face. Pause to generate a slight smile of your own.
- With the intention of being generous, offer this person a phrase such as:
  - "May your happiness grow and be with you always."
  - "May your success continue."
  - "Your joy makes me happy."
- Continue in this way with others who appear to have happiness or success:
  - Someone you like but aren't as close to.
  - A neighbor or acquaintance toward whom you feel neutral.
  - A person you don't know but whose success you admire.

- This practice can also be done not just when meditating but also when you are out among people and noticing their joy or good fortune.
- Imagine yourself encountering someone on the street who seems happy, even though you have no idea why. See yourself as genuinely happy that this person is doing well or has good things. See yourself giving that person a silent offering, such as:
  - "I am so glad for your good fortune."
  - "May you continue to thrive."
  - "Thank you for sharing your joy by showing it."
- Before ending, hold your awareness lightly in the heart center, noticing what is there. If it feels open and warm, be grateful for that. If it does not, that is all right. Accept this time exactly as it has been.

Deep Listening

When someone deeply listens to you,
your bare feet are on the earth
and a beloved land that seemed distant
is now at home within you.

—JOHN FOX

Rick practiced diligently. He was motivated by the changes he was experiencing. "I feel better than I have since I was a kid. I feel lighter, I'm more open and others seem to be responding better to me. I'm more comfortable being around people. Still, I don't know what to say beyond just making conversation. I don't really know how to get close to someone. That's what I *really* want."

Mr. Kanamori, a fourth-grade teacher in Kanazawa, Japan, could teach us all something about deep relationships. He and his class are featured in the moving documentary *Children: Full of Life*, produced by the Japan Broadcasting Corporation (NHK). At the start of the school year, he tells his students that their foremost goal for the year is learning to be happy. One of their primary paths to happiness is learning to share themselves deeply with one another.

He instructs his students to keep notebooks of their personal lives and deepest feelings. During class time, they are given the opportunity to stand before the class and read them aloud to one another. One student, who had just returned from a four-day absence, eagerly marched to the front of the room with his journal in hand to explain why he had been gone. His grandmother had died. He read aloud, sharing his honest feelings as the others listened intently. Many cried. Then some got up and told their own stories, as his reading had unlocked memories of their own losses.

One of the girls told of her father's death when she was just three years old. She had never told any of the other children about it. She hadn't wanted to be different. But after she shared her story, "she was more a part of the class than ever. And now she can talk about her father—and smile."

Mr. Kanamori explains the beauty of this process to the interviewer: "Let people live in your heart. There is no limit on numbers. They tell the stories and everyone shares their feelings. When people really listen . . . they live in your heart forever. That's the great significance of these notebook letters."[3]

Deep listening is a form of compassion that is good both for the one speaking and for those listening. It is made possible by creating a space where the speaker feels safe, protected, and invited to offer his or her truest thoughts and feelings.

Rick recalled his own experience of witnessing the power of

deep listening. It happened when he was a young physician, still in training.

"Thirty years ago," he said, "I was just starting out as a doctor. I worked in a hospital with really sick patients. There was a woman who was clearly dying, but no one ever spoke of it. One night, I was in her room when the charge nurse came in. As she entered, the patient said aloud, 'I'm dying.'

"The charge nurse sat down and asked, 'Are you scared?' That was all she said, but she sat there quietly as if she had no place else to be and nothing more important to do. The dying woman opened up and talked about her fears. I could sense her relief in doing so.

"I realized then that I was scared! I wanted to reassure her, say, 'No, you're not dying.' I wanted to try to make things all right. But what that woman really needed then was someone to just *listen* to her.

"As I watched, it was as if her fear left her and the room was filled with peace. The woman softened. She was ready to let go."

As Rick shared this story, he realized that he *did* know how to be close to another. He had always known—he had just forgotten. He hadn't practiced it for so long that those skills had faded, but they hadn't been lost to him. All he had to do was to keep opening his heart and remember to be present. If he pays attention, he will find plenty of opportunities to be fully present with another.

Mindfulness Practice: The Elements of Deep Listening

- **Presence.** You have been cultivating presence throughout this program. One of its greatest fruits is the ability to be with another with your whole being. As in the story above, there is nowhere else to be, nothing more important to do. You can enhance your presence by turning your awareness to your heart center and inviting your heart to open.

- **Attention.** Again, this has been practiced in each of the meditations. When listening deeply, you are simply placing your attention completely upon the other. If your mind wanders, bring your focus softly back to the person before you. Notice if you are thinking about what you will say or remembering your own similar stories, and let go of your thoughts.

- **See the person's innocence.** Remember how much we are alike, and that we all act unskillfully at times. Release any judgment and open your heart, knowing that this person, like you, is doing the best he or she can at any given moment.

- **See the person's goodness.** One of the most healing things you can do for another is to see his or her basic goodness even when he or she cannot. Trust that the other person doesn't need to be fixed, nor does he or she need your advice. All of us have the wisdom that we need within; it only needs to come into our awareness. See below the surface of the person's words and life to behold his or her resilient, loving nature. It is as if you are holding a great gift for the person until he or she is ready to accept it.

- **Allowing.** None of us can be pressured into speaking our truth. We must be allowed to do so. There is really no action required on your part as the listener, other than to offer a genuine invitation, create a sense of safety, and offer the space and time for the other person. Then trust that the person will speak whatever he or she most needs to hear.

- **Wonder.** If questions arise in response to what another is saying, just hold the questions for a while. Ask only questions that you really wonder about, not those for which you think you know the answer. Your questions best serve when they illuminate the truth for another. You should avoid trying to lead the person to his or her answers. Any truth is richest when we discover it for ourselves.

- **Silence.** Allow for silence—it is where much of the depth resides. Notice if you are tempted to fill a silence with words, and instead return your attention to holding the other with an open heart and a calm mind.

The Soul's Yearning

This is the first, wildest, and wisest thing I know, that the soul exists, and that it is built entirely out of attention.

—MARY OLIVER

Most of us give little attention to what we would consider the "soul" or the "inner voice." Perhaps that is because we don't know how. Yet most of us intuitively know that the soul exists and that it has an important role to play in our degree of happiness and equanimity.

In her poem "The Summer Day" Mary Oliver builds upon the idea of the soul and how to attend to it:

I don't know exactly what a prayer is.
I do know how to pay attention, how to fall down
into the grass, how to kneel down in the grass
how to be idle and blessed, how to stroll through the fields,
which is what I have been doing all day.[4]

Oliver suggests that the sacred can be found by something as simple as holding and watching a grasshopper, by paying attention and being present to that which nature offers us on a summer's day. If we learn how to pay attention, we will see that the sacred is present in nature, in our fellow humans, and in ourselves.

To be at peace with ourselves we must remain connected with our deepest, sacred self and its designs on our lives. It is hard to translate the language of the soul, but we can easily recognize the longing for connection. It is such a key part of being human that we wither and lose heart when we feel disconnected. When we honor that longing for connection and weave it into our lives, our fears and attempts at self-protection fade.

The soul is constantly seeking connection. It is prodding us to be fully engaged in our lives, to know and accept both the highest and lowest aspects of ourselves, to create authentic relationships with others, to be embedded in community, to have meaningful work, to move toward that which we love or long for, to have an experience of the sacred—not just once in a great while, but regularly.

John Tarrant, a Jungian therapist and mindfulness teacher, writes, "It is with our souls that we truly inhabit our lives."[5] Presence, the quality that we have been trying to cultivate with our mindfulness practice, is the natural state of the soul. When we "truly inhabit our lives," when we are most present, the soul reveals itself. Full presence is a reflection of soulfulness.

The soul waits for us to turn our attention toward it. It requires the right conditions to show itself. Think about how you might seek to have an encounter with a wild animal that is wary of humans. You have to approach it indirectly, in a way that is nonthreatening, quiet, almost as if you weren't really there for the purpose of the encounter. You *have* to be fully present. It is like that with the soul. If you stay busy or restless, it will not come forth. If your mind remains unsettled, you will miss it. You must be quiet, patient, and still, inviting it to come forward. And then listen and wait, with all of your attention, so that you can fully inhabit your life.

Mindfulness Practice: Accessing the Wisdom Within

This practice is an invitation to your deepest self to share its wisdom with you. You only need to be still, make the invitation, and then listen intently.

This is done as a guided imagery. A useful image for this practice is that of a seeker going to find a sage. You can picture yourself walking to a mountain lake as the wise older sage sits peacefully beside the lake waiting for you. The sage is really part of yourself—the figure represents your own highest, wisest self. When you are there, you can ask him or her whatever you'd like, and expect that the wisdom you seek will be freely given.

In the middle of the experience, you may choose to write (or draw) in order to express your inner voice. Have everything that you will need set beside you before beginning the meditation. Try to make this a seamless experience so that you stay in a meditative state throughout.

As you write, imagine that your highest self is writing to your ordinary, everyday self. It doesn't have to be anything special or profound. Just let the writing flow, without thinking too much or feeling a need to censor it.

- Get into whatever position you wish, using a chair, cushion, or bench.
- Sit comfortably, back upright but not rigid.
- Check your position and see if you need to shift it to be more comfortable or more upright and alert.
- Begin with a few moments of awareness of the breath, allowing the mind to settle. You may return to the breath as your anchor as you continue with this meditation.
- Picture yourself just as you are at this time in your life.

See yourself walking along a path. You are headed upward, toward a clearing or perhaps a mountain lake. You know that you are going to find your truest, wisest, highest self. And you know that he or she will be there waiting for you.

- Continue to walk along that path, steadily upward, confident of the outcome of your journey.
- See as many details as you can—the width and surface of the path, the hill or mountain in front of you, any surrounding trees, streams, or mountains.
- Hear any sounds: the wind rustling through the trees, the sound of water gently cascading down the hillside, birds singing.
- Notice any smells in the air: pine needles, earth, wildflowers.
- You are getting closer and closer now. In a moment you will be there. Then you will write a message to yourself.
- You have arrived. As you begin writing, imagine that it is the wise sage who is writing. Without censoring, just let your writing flow. Say anything that you think would be helpful to your everyday self. Always the tone will be kind, nonjudging, affirming of yourself.
- What have you learned that you need to be reminded of?
- What might you need in order to meet any challenges before you?
- Offer words of encouragement or comfort.
- Write until you feel you have said all that you need to at this time.
- Now see yourself saying goodbye, taking your leave of this wise being. Know that you can return at any time to ask for further wisdom or advice.
- You are walking away, back down the path. Notice details along the path.

- As you continue walking, notice how you feel. Invite yourself to feel open and secure, confident that you have received just what you needed.
- Now you have come to the end of your journey, for this time at least.
- Return your awareness to the fact that you are sitting. Feel the support from below, and from all around you.
- Place your awareness lightly in the heart center, just noticing what is there. Let yourself feel grateful for however it is.
- Whatever this time has been like for you, accept it fully.

PART THREE

Understand Your Body-Mind

12

The Science of Hope

PEOPLE OFTEN come to the Resilience Training Program after years of futility. They have tried so many things, worked so hard to get better, and still they struggle. They are seeking relief. Many are hoping to get off their medication, or at least to reduce it. Most want to find things that they can do for themselves so that they don't have to rely upon medication or other treatments. All are looking for reason to hope.

My experience has shown that even if you have had a lifetime of struggle, healing is still possible. The chronic effects of stress are potentially *reversible*. I have seen many people reclaim a degree of resilience that they had no longer thought possible. I take inspiration myself in the scientific underpinnings for the Resilience Training Program, some of which I will discuss in this chapter.

I will focus on three areas of recent discovery:

- **Neuroplasticity.** The brain is remarkably resilient and adaptable, making new connections and pruning old ones for as long as we are alive.
- **Neurogenesis.** We keep remaking our brains throughout life by creating brand-new brain cells—and there are things we can do to assist this process.
- **Gene expression.** It is possible to influence the genes that control illnesses such as anxiety or depression.

Each of these topics is a vast and rich body of knowledge, itself worthy of an entire book. While we will only scratch the surface, this science may explain why we can be so successful by taking a multi-pronged approach to recovering from stress and anxiety, even when the usual treatments have failed.

Neuroplasticity: The Brain Is Always Capable of Change

Simply put, the term *neuroplasticity* means that the brain changes in response to new experience. That may not seem like such a revolutionary idea. After all, young children are learning machines—we can practically see their brains changing as we watch them explore, make mistakes, figure things out. Adults, too, are able to learn new things, like a new acquaintance's name or how to use a new cell phone. But what has been discovered in the last few years about neuroscience is indeed revolutionary. Here are just a few highlights:

- The brain is adaptable to a much greater degree than was previously imagined.

- Brain growth doesn't end in childhood—we are able to transform our brain throughout our lives.
- It is even possible to change long-held traits that we think are "just the way we are."

The brain that you have right now has been created, to a large degree, in response to the life that you have led to this point. It has been molded by your experience. More important, the brain you will have in the future depends upon the choices that you make from now on. You can influence the quality of your brain a month, a year, or a decade from now, by what you do today.

It was the great American psychologist William James who, in 1890, described *plasticity* as "the possession of a structure weak enough to yield to an influence, but strong enough not to yield all at once . . . A path once traversed by a nerve-current might be expected to follow the law of most of the paths we know, and to be scooped out and made more permeable than before; and this ought to be repeated with each new passage of the current."[1] In other words, if you create a new dance movement, learn a new song, or even have a new insight, you will create a new neural pathway. If you keep repeating it, the neural connection will be strengthened—that pathway gets "scooped out," becomes better established and easier to traverse. Over time, the path may become so well worn as to develop into a habit. *Anything* that we repeat often enough may become habitual—for good or for ill.

The phrase "use it or lose it" is a good description of what happens to the brain cells, along with a corollary: "What you do use grows stronger." Shortly after James wrote about plasticity, Italian scientists discovered that nerve cells, like muscles, will atrophy if they are not used. They literally shrink. Likewise, they grow bigger if they *are* used, "through the elongation and multiplication of the terminal branches."[2] The end of a neuron is sort of like a fast-growing tree that is stretching out and sending off new shoots in many different directions, and that growth is influenced by how heavily the nerve cell is used.

So individual nerve cells can expand and grow, but how are nerve *circuits* strengthened? It was later discovered that there is a *synapse*, a space between nerve endings where chemicals called neurotransmitters help to convey the signal between one nerve cell and another. An American scientist named Donald Hebb is credited with showing that learning and memory are based upon changes to this nerve synapse. In 1949 he wrote: "The general idea is an old one, that any two cells or systems of cells that are repeatedly active at the same time will tend to become 'associated,' so that activity in one facilitates activity in the other."[3] This theory is summed up in the phrase "nerve cells that fire together wire together." In other words, neurons that are near one another and active at the same time will become functionally connected, forming a neural circuit or network.

In the early 1990s, scientists detailed the process by which enduring changes can occur in these circuits. Known as *long-term potentiation* or LTP, it describes the way that the synapse changes with repeated firing. When it has been "excited" by the chemical messengers, the connection between two nerve cells is strengthened, or potentiated—that is, the synapse learns to fire in this way, and in the future it becomes easier and easier to do so. If the message gets sent a sufficient number of times, the synapse changes in a lasting way and becomes more easily excitable over the long haul—the learning sticks.[4]

But how would that process give someone any hope of real transformation? After all, many people have already spent years trying psychotherapy and self-help techniques, things that offer help but still do not free them from repeated cycles of anxiety and depression.

In fact, many of us strengthen *unhealthy* nerve circuits through repetitive practice. Every time we repeat a fearful or defeatist thought, we strengthen the connections that make it easier to have that thought again. We feed the cycle of fear, keeping the body under continual stress.

But if we can stop reinforcing these patterns by repeated thought, they will gradually weaken. And soon we are able to create new, healthier neural circuits to take the place of the old ones. A new thought, idea, memory, or skill involves the creation of a new neural network in the brain. The more we practice the new pathway, the easier it becomes to keep the new neural network going.

What gives us the capacity to transform ourselves in this seemingly simple way? It is because we possess the will to direct our minds. We can intentionally harness the power of our own thoughts and choose our actions—and thus we can change our brains.

Let me give a straightforward example. Over a decade ago, scientists studied the effect of learning a new motor skill on the brain areas involved with movement. The subjects were instructed to play a five-finger piece on a keyboard connected to a computer, and to do so fluently and in rhythm with a metronome. They practiced two hours per day for five days, and the brain areas corresponding to finger movements were measured before and after. Sure enough, those motor areas grew significantly—that's not too surprising, knowing that nerve cells grow with use. But what was remarkable about this experiment was that the researchers had another group do the practice *only in their minds*: they didn't actually move their fingers, they just *imagined* their fingers moving. And they had a similar change in their brains! Their neural circuits were stimulated and grew—solely in response to thought.[5]

That's pretty amazing, and it's nice to know that mental rehearsal may actually improve motor skills. Athletes who spend time imagining themselves doing a perfect gymnastics routine or sinking a three-point shot may indeed perform better as a result. But what of the stress response and the fear circuitry—can those also be altered at will, through engaging the mind in a novel way?

If you have ever been caught in a cycle of anxious thinking, you know that it is hard to will yourself out of it, especially in the heat of the moment. But it *is* possible, given enough time and practice. In fact, fear conditioning, where a stimulus (such as speaking in front of a group) is paired with the fear response, is a learned behavior. Remember Pavlov's dog, who learned to salivate each time a bell was rung because that bell had been paired with food? We're no different. We learn to associate cues in our environment with fear, because at one time such a cue occurred just before or during a fearful experience. But what can be learned can also be unlearned. Fear can be extinguished, and there is ample evidence to prove it.

For example, researchers at UCLA showed that the fear circuit, which gets stuck in the on position in active obsessive-compulsive disorder, calmed down with successful behavioral treatment involving mindfulness practices.[6] Teaching mindfulness meditation to sufferers of OCD gave them the power to turn off the stuck switch, effectively rewiring their own brains.[7] Other studies have found a similar phenomenon in post-traumatic stress disorder, where brain scanning showed that by learning to work with their minds, study participants were able to quiet their overly active amygdala.[8]

Similarly, a study on phobias (the most common of all psychiatric conditions) revealed a dramatic change after cognitive-behavior therapy. In this case, they worked with twelve women with a spider phobia. Every one of them responded to treatment and were able afterward to do increasingly difficult tasks: touch pictures of spiders, a TV screen showing moving spiders, and eventually even a living spider— and their fear circuitry, measured by fMRI, remained as calm as in the normal controls. The researchers concluded that "changes made at the mind level, within a psychotherapeutic context, are able to functionally 'rewire' the brain . . . In other words, 'change the mind and you change the brain.'"[9]

Not only can you free yourself from a particular illness by training your mind, but also it is possible to transform a long-held unhealthy trait into a more resilient one. Richard Davidson, at the University of Wisconsin, has studied affective style (the different ways that we respond emotionally to challenges) and the related concept of the emotional set point (the underlying, baseline mood that we return to after we've had an emotional reaction). Both of these traits have long been assumed to be unchangeable, and each has a lot to do with resilience.

Highly resilient people tend to be less emotionally reactive. It's not that they don't have negative emotions—they do. But their emotional reaction is not as intense and is less harmful to them, and they recover more quickly from it. When they do recover, they return to a more positive baseline mood. We all want to be more resilient, but isn't this just "how we're wired"? Is it really possible to change these traits, to *learn* to have a more resilient affective style?

Dr. Davidson and his colleagues have shown that there is an asymmetry in the prefrontal cortex reflecting our affective style. When there is more activity in the right side of the prefrontal cortex, it correlates with negative emotions such as worry, sadness, and anger. If the left side is more active, we tend to be in a positive emotional state, with a sense of well-being, enthusiasm, even joy.[10] Developing greater resilience, then, should show up as a shift in the relative activity between the two sides of the prefrontal cortex: the left side ought to become more active as the right side calms down. In fact, that happened with a group that practiced mindfulness meditation for eight weeks. They had greater activity in the left side, reported a stronger sense of well-being, and even showed a positive change in immune system function, as measured by influenza antibody titers. Those who had the most activity in the left prefrontal cortex had the strongest immune system response, suggesting a connection between overall well-being and the health of the immune system.[11]

But the scientists had an even more ambitious study in mind. Can we be more calm, happy, or compassionate not just in the short term but in an enduring way? After much coaxing, they convinced Buddhist monks, experts in meditation, to be studied using fMRI scans. What they found was an astounding shift in the monks' degree of left frontal activity that far surpassed anything seen before. Presumably that was an effect of the monks' long-term mental training. Yet even novices to meditation, when given some instruction on how to do a compassion practice, showed a shift to stronger activity on the left side of the prefrontal cortex and a greater sense of well-being. It is possible to make ourselves happier, calmer, and more resilient—just by doing inner work![12]

Neurogenesis: You Can Build a New Brain

Whereas neuroplasticity involves primarily strengthening or weakening the connections between existing neurons, there is another exciting discovery that gives further hope to anyone caught in an unhealthy long-term pattern. The brain is able to create new neurons, to grow and heal itself. And that possibility remains with us not just when we are young but throughout our lives.

That is not what I learned in my training. Like most physicians, I learned that the brain, once developed, remains more or less as is for the remainder of our lives. Whereas the rest of the body is continually changing, repairing itself and rebuilding, we believed that the brain is more of a stable, unchanging entity. We are able to learn new things and make new connections, but only within the parameters given us at birth, or shortly thereafter. We are born with a certain number of brain cells, the brain assembles itself in the first few years of life, and the best we can do after that is to maintain as much function as possible. Over the course of our lives, brain cells gradually die off—a process hastened by exposure to toxins such as alcohol or petrochemicals, or by brain injury or strokes. After a neuron had died, we believed, it could never grow back. Once a function was lost, we assumed that it could never be recovered.

To some extent, that is all true. Your brain can indeed be damaged beyond repair, toxins do destroy brain cells, and neurons do die as we age. But our assumptions have been challenged in dramatic ways, and we now know that there are stem cells in the brain that are capable of creating new, healthy brain cells and restoring normal function to an amazing degree—throughout our lives.

The myth that new brain growth stopped after early development was first shattered by studies on songbirds, of all things. A paper came out in 1983 describing how female canaries had produced many new neurons in the part of the brain involved with song control. This was unusual because these were *adult* birds, and the researchers concluded that the "neurogenesis we have observed in the adult brain is both provocative and reassuring of the plasticity that may reside in adult nervous systems."[13]

The new cell growth was documented by injecting a radioactive material into the birds that would later become woven into their DNA. But it would only show up in the DNA of new cells that were created *after* the injection. Proving this required sacrificing the animals to examine their brain tissue. Obviously, scientists could not repeat this study in humans, so no one knew whether this new cell growth occurred in people, too. But fifteen years later, Swedish researchers came upon the idea of studying patients who were in the end stages of terminal cancer. With their permission, they were injected with the same radioactive material as the songbirds, and after they died their brains were examined. In the hippocampus (the memory center) of these patients, they found new cells sprouting from neuronal stem cells at an amazing rate. This study showed, for the first time ever, that there was new cell growth in the adult human brain—and this occurred in terminally ill people who were in their fifties, sixties, and seventies, right up until the time of death![14]

Proving that we keep growing new brain cells raises an obvious question: can we improve this new cell growth, and if so, how? It turns out that there are numerous chemical growth factors, including several that act in the nervous system, where they are known as *neurotrophins*. Brain-derived neurotrophic factor, or BDNF, has perhaps received the most attention. BDNF appears to be most active in the hippocampus (and to a lesser degree the cortex), where it promotes the growth of new cells, improves memory and learning, and enhances the survival of existing neurons. These neurotrophins also influence the process of neuroplasticity, controlling where new nerve branches go, pruning the old, unused ones, and deciding which neurons to connect with others in a neural circuit.[15]

Low levels of BDNF have been linked to many diseases, including depression and anxiety, Alzheimer's, and Parkinson's disease, among others.[16] What do all of these chronic conditions have in common? All are related to prolonged stress and elevated cortisol levels. BDNF gives us crucial protection against the effects of cortisol—it helps the neurons survive—as well as increasing the number of new cells created. Interestingly, if a newly created neuron doesn't connect with other neurons soon after it is born, it will shrivel up and die. The most important factor in their early survival is that they become connected to other cells. In fact, this may explain how stress shrinks the hippocampus—because long-term exposure to cortisol reduces the ability of BDNF to foster those crucial neural connections.[17]

I think of BDNF and other neurotrophins as the brain's master gardeners. Naturally, we want to give these gardeners the tools they need—fertilizer, pruning shears, and rich soil—so that our neurons remain healthy and plentiful as we age. Factors that can help to do just that include enriched learning environments, exercise, a healthy diet, good levels of serotonin, and social connection.

Enriched Learning Environments: Helping Cells Connect

The early research on neuroplasticity by Hebb and others showed that having new experiences could result in a greater capacity to learn. Hebb first came upon this insight by accident. He began taking some of his laboratory rats home as pets, and noticed that they became more curious and adept at learning than the rats that remained caged in the lab.[18]

More rigorous studies conducted in the 1960s showed that rats who were given an enriched environment—that is, they were housed in groups rather than alone, and were given plenty of toys to play with—were able to solve mazes better than their more deprived mates.[19] In fact, studies showed that mice developed bigger brains because their enriched environments led to greater neurogenesis.[20] And these new brain cells were produced not just in young animals but in older mice as well.[21]

Exercise: Boosting BDNF Levels

One of the toys available in the mice's enriched environment was a treadmill, and when given the opportunity, the mice spent hours on the treadmill each day. It turns out that exercise is one of the most potent ways to elevate levels of BDNF and create greater production of new cells. The mice that had the opportunity to run had twice as many new neurons as those that couldn't.[22]

The benefits of exercise on BDNF begin quickly (within two to three days) and last a long time (several weeks at least). And they occur in older brains as well as in younger ones, although perhaps in slightly different areas of the hippocampus.[23] Not only did the exercised mice produce more neurons, but those new cells were also healthier, had more branches coming off the ends, and were better prepared to connect to other cells.[24] Just what a master gardener likes to see—lots of healthy new growth!

Since these discoveries, researchers have tried to clarify what kind of exercise, and how much, has the greatest effect on BDNF. We still don't have a definitive answer, but some clues are beginning to emerge suggesting that low-level, nonstrenuous exercise may be best at boosting BDNF, at least in the long term.[25] It seems that short bursts of intense exercise elevate BDNF, but only for a brief time, and then levels drop again. In fact, there appears to be an inverse relationship between BDNF levels at rest and a person's level of cardiovascular fitness: the fitter someone is, the lower his or her resting levels of BDNF.[26]

My take on this finding is that it reflects the system as it is supposed to work in healthy people. Intense exercise is a lot like activating the fight-or-flight mechanism—it creates a short-term stress. In response to that stress, BDNF levels rise to activate the hippocampus and generate new learning. Remember, if there were an actual threat, it would be helpful to create new memories in order to avoid a similar situation in the future. Within just a few minutes after the stress has subsided, those memories should have been encoded with the help of BDNF. Cortisol levels then rise to shut down the hippocampus, consolidate the learning, and put the system back to a normal resting level.

That theory seems consistent with a study done of healthy male athletes, measuring their BDNF and cortisol levels before and after a mild ten-minute aerobic warm-up, and then again after exercising them to exhaustion. They found that BDNF did not change during the warm-up period, but it did increase at the point of exhaustion and then returned to baseline within a few minutes. Cortisol levels, on the other hand, were increased ten to fifteen minutes after exercise and took longer to return to baseline than did BDNF.[27] This simply reflects the normal role of cortisol in the stress cycle.

I believe that it is good for us to be stressed once in a while, especially if we do so voluntarily through occasional vigorous exercise. Still, if you just don't like vigorous exercise, you should take heart from the research. Moving your body at all, even with occasional light exercise, may improve the health of your brain and protect you from stress, anxiety, depression, and age-related decline.

Remember, though, that for cells to survive and become functional, they have to connect to other neurons soon after they are produced or they will die. In order for that connecting to occur, there needs to be more than the birth of new cells—there also has to be new learning. The more learning that occurs, and the greater the effort put into it, the greater the number of neurons that are likely to survive. So fitness works hand in hand with a rich learning environment—physical exercise helps create new brain cells, while mental exercise helps those newborn cells connect and thrive.

Diet: Protecting the New Cells

Exercise is not the only physical factor that encourages new cell growth. The environment in which the new cells are created, the degree to which there is healthy "soil" for these new cells to take root, is likewise important. In that regard, diet is showing itself to be another important element for high BDNF function and a healthy brain.

The earliest research on diet and BDNF, published just a few years ago, studied the effect of dietary restriction on neurogenesis. It was already known that rats that were placed on a low-calorie diet were relatively protected from age-related learning and memory problems, and the researchers wondered if that protection was related to BDNF and neurogenesis. In fact, they found a significant increase of BDNF and new cells in the hippocampus when the rats were calorie restricted, mostly because the new cells had a much better chance of surviving.[28]

I believe that this finding has to do with there being less oxidative stress when calories are restricted. Less oxidation because of fewer calories consumed means that there are fewer harmful free radicals. It would then make sense that protecting against the effects of oxidation, as the antioxidants are meant to do, could offer a similar benefit.

Research coming out in the past couple of years supports this hypothesis. Fruits and vegetables, which are rich in phytonutrients, have been shown to aid in reversing age-related deficits in memory and learning. In one study, aging animals' diets were supplemented with blueberries, a fruit known to be high in flavonoids, which provide potent antioxidant protection. Within three weeks, the animals showed a significant improvement in memory and increased activity of BDNF in the hippocampus.[29] And in a study with humans, researchers found that those who ate more fresh fruit (at least five or six times per week) had higher levels of BDNF.[30] Indeed, antioxidants appear to aid in healthy neurogenesis.

The third dietary factor identified so far with an impact on BDNF is omega-3 fatty acids. Omega-3s have a number of positive effects on brain function, including protection against cell death. Researchers looked at whether a diet high in omega-3 fats could protect rats from brain injury. They induced a mild injury from oxidative stress. The rats that did not have omega-3 in their diets had lower levels of BDNF, which affected their memory after the injury—they were less capable of learning a water maze afterward. Remarkably, omega-3 supplementation counteracted *all* of the effects of the injury, reducing oxidative damage, normalizing BDNF levels, and preserving the animals' learning ability.[31] This gives me even more reason to think that eating healthy amounts of omega-3 fats may be one of the best things that you can do for your brain.

Serotonin and BDNF: A Dynamic Duo in Neurogenesis

Another great thing for the brain is maintaining a healthy level of serotonin. Not only is it important for mood and anxiety; serotonin also gives BDNF a boost. The two chemicals are partners: serotonin helps regulate neuroplasticity and neurogenesis, while BDNF improves the growth and survival of serotonin neurons.[32] Anything that improves serotonin function, such as diet, exercise, sleep, even antidepressants, may in turn enhance the effects of BDNF.[33]

Social Connection: Harnessing the Power to Heal

Before leaving the topic of neurogenesis, I want to describe one more study that sheds light on what is most important to the brain, and therefore to our ability to respond well to stress and anxiety. This study set out to compare several of the key factors that regulate BDNF in the aging brain: moderate exercise, dietary restriction, and an enriched environment, defined here as living in a group of four animals, as opposed to those who lived in isolation. The researchers looked at both young and old rats and found that, in general, the younger rats had higher levels of BDNF—no surprise there. But their overall conclusions *were* surprising.

They found that, for the older animals, the highest levels of BDNF by far were in those that lived in groups, even though they were sedentary and were given access to as much food as they wanted. Even more remarkable, their levels were even higher than in the young baseline group. This suggests that we receive great protection from stress and aging through positive social connection.[34] This is a theme that recurs over and over again in the literature on resilience. Truly, we are meant to be connected with others.

Genetic Expression: Genes Don't Change—or Do They?

The genetic information that we have received from our parents is wrapped up nicely in our DNA, the double helix that by now is familiar to us all. Genes carry information from one generation to the next, instructing the body as to how to build itself, beginning with the first cell division and continuing for the rest of our lives. DNA also conveys the traits, skills, and attributes that largely make us who we are. But what, really, does it do? How does DNA translate its information into our bodies and brains, and can that process be altered? Are genes immutable, so that whatever we have inherited binds us irrevocably to our forebears, for better or worse?

The job of DNA, in essence, is to give instructions to the machinery of the cells for the building of proteins. Those proteins not only give us our physical structure but also make possible the millions of different functions that the body carries out every day. In addition to building muscle and sinew, our DNA directs the production of all the various chemical messengers, enzymes, and hormones—the stuff that makes our bodies run. All are made up of proteins constructed by the blueprint that DNA provides.

There is an intermediary in this production process called *messenger RNA* (mRNA) that takes the blueprints from DNA and brings them to the factory floor in the cell so that just the right protein sequence is produced. This translation process is highly variable— mRNA does not receive the same instructions from DNA each time the blueprint is delivered. But if the DNA sequence is unchanging, how is it possible that it can give out different messages?

It is true that the DNA sequence that you inherited from your parents at the moment of conception is fixed and will remain as is throughout your life, barring a genetic mutation. That fixed sequence is known as your *genotype*, and it sets the parameters for your good health, as well as your relative risk for developing disease. But how your genes are *expressed*—whether and how they show up in your life—is actually quite variable. The expression of genes is called the *phenotype*, and it is influenced by a host of different factors, many of them environmental. This is why an illness such as anxiety, depression, or type 2 diabetes may become a reality for one member of a pair of identical twins but not for the other, even though both have exactly the same genetic information encoded in their DNA. As they get older, in fact, identical twins become more and more different from each other in the expression of their genes. Why is that? It is because their environments become more and more variable over time.[35]

So what are these environmental factors that influence genetic expression, and what can we do about them? As you can see, there are several on this list that are part of the Resilience Training Program:

- Physical factors such as exercise.
- Chemical exposures, including well-known factors such as alcohol or tobacco, but also endocrine disrupters such as those found in plastics or chemical fertilizers. And there are positive modifiers, too, such as the healthy phytonutrients in fruits and vegetables.
- Mental or emotional factors, such as the effects of long-term stress or, on the other hand, the cultivating of positive emotions, can also change gene expression.

The name given to these changes in gene expression is *epigenetics*, and the study of it is very new. It seems that the expression of genes allows us to "record" information in our bodies so that we can respond to changes in our environment without altering our basic gene sequence. If there is a change in the availability of food, for example, it would be helpful to turn some genes on and others off, so that we can respond to that change until things return to normal.

How is this feat accomplished? There is a sophisticated code, known as the *histone code*, that directs the decisions as to which parts of the DNA sequence are transcribed into mRNA and which are not. There are several means by which to change the histone code, including a recently discovered regulator of this process called microRNA.[36] Another involves methylation, a process by which access to the gene sequence is either allowed or denied. Many genes can be "marked" by having a methyl molecule added to a particular site on the DNA strand, and this marking turns that gene on or off. Genes that are methylated do not get transcribed into mRNA—access to that part of the gene sequence is blocked, so they are effectively silenced.[37] But it is also possible to change those markings. Enzymes can remove the methyl molecule through a process called demethylation, reopening access to that particular part of the gene. This whole process is very dynamic, allowing genes to be turned on or turned off as circumstances change.

For example, there is a gene in a certain strain of mice that, when activated, results in them developing yellowish fur, becoming obese, and acquiring the illnesses that come with obesity, such as hypertension and diabetes. This gene can be turned off by feeding the mothers a diet high in folate and vitamin B_{12} while they are pregnant. The B vitamins act as "methyl donors" and fill the open sites in the gene, thereby silencing the gene. Their offspring are darker-colored, lean, and healthy.[38]

Another study supporting this hypothesis was done with sheep. When B_{12} and folate were taken out of ewes' diets just briefly, near the time of conception, their offspring became overweight as adults, with high blood pressure and insulin resistance. This was also caused by changes in methylation at the gene level.[39]

In humans, too, these factors come into play. You may know that pregnant women are prescribed prenatal vitamins high in folate and B vitamins, among other nutrients. In part, this is meant to reduce birth defects, in which the methylation process is again important.

Another recent discovery found that there is a wide spectrum of activity of an enzyme known as MTHF reductase. In some people this enzyme is deficient, effectively reducing their folate levels. This impairs their DNA methylation, perhaps making them more susceptible to illnesses such as anxiety or depression.[40]

The body-mind connection can also influence gene expression. When scientists do animal studies on anxiety, they remove infant rats from their mothers and siblings and place them in a separate cage. This creates isolation distress, a condition remarkably similar to human anxiety states. These infants are then returned to their families a few minutes later. There are some mothers who are naturally more nurturing than others, and they respond by licking and grooming their frightened infants. These attentive mothers cuddle their babies as a means of soothing their distress. But there are other mothers that provide little, if any, of this nurturance, leaving their infants to fend for themselves. When they grow up, which group do you think does better at handling stress?

It may come as little surprise that, when they reach adulthood, the rats that were better soothed and nurtured show fewer signs of fearfulness and anxiety. Their stress response system is less reactive. Sure, they still get stressed when they feel threatened, and their cortisol levels go up—but their stress response quickly subsides. There's more, though—rats that had been distressed as babies and then were adequately soothed did better than those that were never distressed in the first place. When they became stressed as adults, the rats that had never gone through this isolation distress became more fearful and their cortisol levels took much longer to come back down.[41] There is something helpful, it seems, about being stressed and then soothed immediately afterward.

Later it was shown that this damping of the stress response comes about through changing gene expression. The soothing maternal behavior altered the glucocorticoid receptor gene. This helped the better-nurtured mice to develop a more efficient cortisol feedback loop. Their environment, which included a nurturing mother, turned on the gene that produced cortisol receptors, so the receptors became more numerous. Those rats were then able to shut down their cortisol production much more quickly than the others—a healthier pattern that stayed with them into adulthood.[42]

These traits, programmed early in life, are enduring—but not necessarily permanent. They can be changed later in life by factors that alter DNA methylation. In one study, anxious adult rats were made calmer by injecting a substance that alters methylation. Afterward, they became much less reactive to stress, just like those who had been well nurtured as infants.[43]

This is still a new science, and much of the research has been done on animals. But there are intriguing findings cropping up in humans, too. There was a recent study of the effects of laughter on type 2 diabetes. The subjects' blood glucose was measured before and after a meal, and the researchers found that laughter slowed the rise in blood sugar—a good thing for diabetics. But they also looked at more than eighteen thousand genes to see which ones were upregulated—that is, which were turned on—by laughter. Interestingly, only twenty-three genes were turned on, and none of them was directly involved with regulating blood glucose. It was the dopamine D4 receptor gene that had this positive impact on blood sugar. Dopamine, you may recall, is one of the key neurotransmitters involved with mood, mental focus, and pleasure—and a gene that regulated it was turned on by laughing.[44]

Another study looked at the effects of the relaxation response, a well-established body-mind training that helps turn off the stress response. Meditation and breathing techniques are examples of ways to elicit the relaxation response, though there are many others. In this study, they had three groups with about twenty participants each: one set of long-term practitioners of the relaxation response, one group that received eight weeks of training in the technique, and a control group. They found that both of the groups that practiced the relaxation response had a significantly positive change in the expression of genes related to stress. Many of the genes that are usually turned on by stress were turned off instead, which protected the cells in the face of oxidative stress.[45]

As we go through life, we are exposed to more and more environmental challenges, ranging from chemical exposures to job stresses to loss of loved ones. And as we age, the methylation marking system becomes more and more prone to error, leaving open a greater possibility of our developing certain diseases.[46] For good or for ill, our environment becomes relatively more important as the influence of our original DNA sequence diminishes over time.

Early life exposures to dietary and environmental factors set up important, long-standing patterns, but those early patterns can be altered. It is important to remember that, in fact, there are positive influences on genes and health, and that seemingly "soft" interventions, such as soothing touch, relaxing the mind, or experiencing a good feeling, can impact something as biological as gene expression. Your DNA and how it becomes manifest is a dynamic, ever-changing system. It is my hope that this book helps you in every way possible to move that genetic expression in a positive direction.

Afterword

The Call to Courage

Caretake this moment. Immerse yourself in its particulars.
It is time to really live; to fully inhabit the situation you happen to be in now.
You are not some disinterested bystander.

—EPICTETUS

EVERY TIME I meet with people who are struggling with their fears, really wrestling with them, I am struck by the courage that they show. It is not easy to face each day like this, to "wake up empty and scared," as Rumi put, and then to go forth and try to really live.

Yet that is our task, isn't it? We are all seeking to inhabit our lives more fully, whatever is before us, no matter the particulars.

Epictetus went on to say: "As concerns the art of living, the material is your own life. No great thing is created suddenly. There must be time."[1] Courage is not just the absence of fear. It is an enlivened state that goes beyond thought, beyond emotion, beyond even spiritual practice. Fear and anxiety may stop us from taking action, even that which the soul longs for. Fear may stop us for a while, but we can

253

remember that "no great thing is created suddenly"—and that includes the greatness of our own lives.

Courage allows us to be drawn by purpose and meaning. By attending to the material of your own life, you can find the courage to face the particulars of your life and to take committed and effective action, whether fear is present or not. That courage does not really need to be found. It already resides in you.

> *When your fears surrender to your strengths,*
> *You will begin to experience*
> *That all existence*
> *Is a teeming sea of infinite life.*[2]
>
> —Hafiz

When your fears surrender to your strengths, when you awaken to who you really are, when you acknowledge what you are really capable of, when you claim the courage and resilience that are your nature—then you will calmly experience how good it is to be in this world.

Acknowledgments

I HAVE a deep sense of gratitude to the many people who have aided in the birthing of *The Chemistry of Calm*. It began with my editor at Simon & Schuster, Michelle Howry, whose idea first sparked the book, and whose steady, graceful guidance has made this process seem to flow so seamlessly. My literary agent, Janis Vallely, has provided such encouragement and support along with a uniquely discerning eye for writing. I can't believe my good fortune in having Michelle and Janis on my team.

I have had a unique opportunity to put my ideas into practice at one of the best integrative medical centers in the country—the Penny George Institute for Health and Healing. I am forever grateful to Penny George and the George Family Foundation for their unfailing support, and to Lori Knutson, director of the Institute, for being such a visionary guide for the Resilience Training Program. I am also blessed to work with a truly great team: Carolyn Denton, our brilliant integrative nutritionist; Sue Masemer, a gifted exercise physiologist and incredibly supportive manager; and the staff at the LiveWell Fitness Center, including Gail Ericson, Jeannie Paris, and Patty DeClercq.

Special thanks go to my teaching colleagues and long-term work partners, Sandra Kacher and Susan Bourgerie. We have spent many hours together honing the ideas that have formed the approach described in this book. Sandy and Susan are not only wonderful collaborators, but also great friends who embody the principles that we teach.

I received a vast amount of help in the research for this book from Victoria Wirtz, whose commitment to this work is an inspiration. There were several others who, like Victoria, read and commented on the chapters as they emerged, including Jennifer Blair, Jan Swanson, Sue Towey, Jamie Loso, and Rosemary Camilleri. The effort and thoughtfulness that they put into this work is a reflection of their own generous spirits, and I am so grateful for their ongoing friendship.

I could not have written this book without the strength, love, and support of my wife, Jane Blockhus, and my sons, Eric and Mark. Thank you for the many blessings that you give so freely.

Finally, I want to thank the patients whose courage and grace in the face of suffering and whose willingness to move toward wholeness give such beautiful expression to this human experience.

Notes

Chapter 1: The Promise of Tranquility

1. R. C. Kessler et al., "Lifetime Prevalence and Age-of-Onset Distributions of *DSM-IV* Disorders in the National Comorbidity Survey Replication," *Archives of General Psychiatry* 62, no. 6 (June 2005): 593–602.

2. R. L. DuPont et al., "Economic Costs of Anxiety Disorders," *Anxiety* 2 (2006): 167–172.

3. A. Gomez-Caminero et al., "Does Panic Disorder Increase the Risk of Coronary Heart Disease? A Cohort Study of a National Managed Care Database," *Psychosomatic Medicine* 67 (2005): 688–691.

4. J. Stein et al., "Environmental Threats to Healthy Aging: With a Closer Look at Alzheimer's and Parkinson's Diseases," report by the Greater Boston Physicians for Social Responsibility and Science and Environmental Health Network, 2008.

5. S. M. Grundy et al., "Definition of Metabolic Syndrome," *Circulation* 109 (2004): 433–438.

6. M. Timonen et al., "Insulin Resistance and Depressive Symptoms in Young Adult Males: Findings from Finnish Military Conscripts," *Psychosomatic Medicine* 69, no. 8 (2007): 723–728.

7. K. Yaffe et al., "The Metabolic Syndrome, Inflammation and Risk of Cognitive Decline," *Journal of the American Medical Association* 292, no. 18 (2004): 2237–2242.

8. R. M. Sapolsky, "Stress, Health and Coping," presentation at the American Association for the Advancement of Science, February 5, 2007. Quoted in "Why Do Humans and Primates Get More Stress-Related Diseases than Other Animals?" *ScienceDaily*, Stanford University (February 25, 2007), www.sciencedaily.com/releases/2007/02/070218134333.htm.

Chapter 2: A Brief History of Anxiety

1. M. Lewis and J. M. Haviland-Jones, eds., *Handbook of Emotions*, 2nd edition (New York: Guilford Press, 2000).
2. R. L. M. Dunbar and L. Barrett, eds., *The Oxford Handbook of Evolutionary Psychology* (Oxford: Oxford University Press, 2007).
3. R. A. Gabriel, *No More Heroes: Madness and Psychiatry In War* (New York: Hill and Wang, 1987).
4. J. L. Herman, *Trauma and Recovery* (New York: Basic Books, 1997).
5. Gabriel, *No More Heroes*.
6. Herman, *Trauma and Recovery*.
7. G. S. Patton and M. Blumenson, *The Patton Papers* (New York: Da Capo Press, 1996).
8. Gabriel, *No More Heroes*.
9. J. W. Appel and G. W. Beebe, "Preventive Psychiatry: An Epidemiologic Approach," *Journal of the American Medical Association* 131 (1946): 1469–1475.
10. B. P. Dohrenwend et al., "The Psychological Risks of Vietnam for U.S. Veterans: A Revisit with New Data and Methods," *Science* 313, no. 5789 (August 18, 2006): 979–982.
11. J. A. Boscarino, "Posttraumatic Stress Disorder and Mortality Among U.S. Army Veterans 30 Years After Military Service," *Annals of Epidemiology* 16, no. 4 (April 2006): 248–256.
12. "The Psychological Needs of U.S. Military Service Members and Their Families." American Psychological Association, February 25, 2007.
13. M. H. Stone, *Healing the Mind: A History of Psychiatry from Antiquity to the Present* (New York: Norton, 1997).
14. R. Porter, *Medicine: A History of Healing: Ancient Traditions to Modern Practices* (New York: Ivy Press, 1997).
15. Herman, *Trauma and Recovery*.
16. S. Freud, *Studies on Hysteria* (New York: Basic Books, 2000).
17. W. James, quoted in Herman, *Trauma and Recovery*.
18. W. B. Cannon, "The Interrelations of Emotions as Suggested by Recent Physiological Researches," *American Journal of Psychology* 25, no. 2 (April 1914): 256–282.
19. R. M. Sapolsky, *Why Zebras Don't Get Ulcers*, 3rd edition (New York: Macmillan, 2004).
20. E. Shorter, *A History of Psychiatry: From the Era of the Asylum to the Age of Prozac* (New York: Wiley, 1997).
21. Ibid.
22. C. M. Callahan and G. E. Barros, *Reinventing Depression* (Oxford: Oxford University Press, 2005).
23. Centers for Disease Control and Prevention, *Health, United States*, U.S. Department of Health and Human Services, 2007.

24. "What's in a Pill?" *Psychology Today* (May 2002): 4; as quoted in R. Kadison, *College of the Overwhelmed* (San Francisco: Jossey-Bass, 2004).

25. Center for Drug Evaluation and Research, "Suicidality in Children and Adolescents Being Treated with Antidepressant Medications," U.S. Food and Drug Administration, October 15, 2004.

26. S. W. Keith et al, "Putative Contributors to the Secular Increase in Obesity: Exploring the Roads Less Travelled," *International Journal of Obesity* 30 (June 2006): 1585–1594; R. R. Rubin, "Depression Symptoms, Antidepressant Medicine Use and Risk of Developing Diabetes in Diabetes Prevention Programs," *American Diabetes Association Scientific Sessions,* June 9–13, 2006, Abstract 869-P; S. J. Diem et al, "Use of Antidepressants and Rates of Hip Bone Loss in Older Women: The Study of Osteoporotic Fractures," *Archives of Internal Medicine* 167, no. 12 (2007): 1240–1245; E. M. Haney et al, "Association of Low Bone Mineral Density with Selective Serotonin Reuptake Inhibitor Use by Older Men," *Archives of Internal Medicine* 167, no. 12 (2007): 1246–1251.

Chapter 3: The Roots of Resilience

1. E. A. Holmes et al., "Can Playing the Computer Game 'Tetris' Reduce the Build-up of Flashbacks for Trauma? A Proposal from Cognitive Science," *PLoS ONE* 4, vol. 1 (January 7, 2009): e4153.

Chapter 4: Balance Your Brain Chemistry

1. M. Pollan, "Unhappy Meals," *New York Times Magazine,* January 28, 2007.

2. R. J. Colman, R. M. Anderson, et al., "Caloric Restriction Delays Disease Onset and Mortality in Rhesus Monkeys," *Science* 325, no. 5937 (July 10, 2009): 201–204.

3. J. Stein et al., "Environmental Threats to Healthy Aging: With a Closer Look at Alzheimer's and Parkinson's Diseases," report by the Greater Boston Area Physicians for Social Responsibility and Science and Environmental Health Network, 2008.

4. Pollan, "Unhappy Meals."

5. A. Rubio-Tapia et al., "Increased Prevalence and Mortality in Undiagnosed Celiac Disease," *Gastroenterology* 137, no. 1 (July 2009): 88–93.

6. J. Marcotti, "Science Confirms Increase in Wheat Gluten Disorder," *Star Tribune,* July 1, 2009.

7. Environmental Working Group, *Shopper's Guide to Pesticides,* March 10, 2009, www.foodnews.org.

8. Environmental Working Group, "Fish Safety Alert," September 30, 2002, http://www.ewg.org/node/15021.

9. Nutrient Data Laboratory, "Oxygen Radical Absorption Capacity (ORAC) of Selected Foods—2007," U.S. Department of Agriculture, November 2007, www.ars.usda.gov/SP2UserFiles/Place/12354500/Data/ORAC/ORAC07.pdf.

10. G. A. Bray et al., "Consumption of High-Fructose Corn Syrup in Beverages May Play a Role in the Epidemic of Obesity," *American Journal of Clinical Nutrition* 79 (2004): 537–543.

11. A.P. Simopoulos, "Overview of Evolutionary Aspects of Omega-3 Fatty Acids in Diet," *World Review of Nutrition and Dietetics* 83 (1998): 1–11.

12. www.slowfood.com/about_us/eng/taste_education.lasso.

13. P. J. Stover and M. A. Caudill, "Genetic and Epigenetic Contributions to Human Nutrition and Health: Managing Genome-Diet Interactions," *Journal of the American Dietetic Association* 108 (2008): 1480–1487.

Chapter 5: Balance Your Brain Chemistry (Continued)

1. B. Hassel and R. Dingledine, "Glutamate," in G. J. Siegel et al., eds., *Basic Neurochemistry: Molecular, Cellular and Medical Aspects* (Burlington, MA: Elsevier Academic Press, 2006).

2. A.H. Kim et al., "Blocking Excitotoxicity," in F. W. Marcoux and D. W. Choi, eds., *CNS Neuroprotection* (New York: Springer, 2002): 3–36.

3. L. S. Krimer et al., "Dopaminergic Regulation of Cerebral Cortical Microcirculation," *Nature Neuroscience* 1 (1998): 286–289.

4. M. Wichers and M. Maes, "The Psychoneuroimmuno-Pathophysiology of Cytokine Induced Depression in Humans," *International Journal of Neuropsychopharmacology* 5 (2002): 375–438.

5. R. Peled et al., "Breast Cancer, Psychological Distress and Life Events Among Young Women," *BMC Cancer* 8 (2008): 245.

6. H. A. Alhaj, A. E. Massey, et al., "Effects of DHEA Administration on Episodic Memory, Cortisol and Mood in Healthy Young Men: A Double-Blind, Placebo-Controlled Study," *Psychopharmacology* 188, no. 4 (2006): 541–551.

7. M. L. Neuhouser et al., "Multivitamin Use and Risk of Cancer and Cardiovascular Disease in the Women's Health Initiative Cohorts," *Archives of Internal Medicine* 169, no. 3 (2009): 293–304.

8. J. Liu et al, "DNA Methylation Affects Cell Proliferation, Cortisol Secretion and Steroidogenic Gene Expression in Human Adrenocortical NCI-H295R Cells," *Journal of Molecular Endocrinology* 33 (2004): 651–662.

9. T. Bottiglieri et al., "Homocysteine, Folate, Methylation and Monoamine Metabolism in Depression," *Journal of Neurology, Neurosurgery and Psychiatry* 69 (2000): 228–232.

10. J. Lombard, "Neurobiology of Mood and Cognition: Strategies and Protocols of Neurotransmitter Balance," presented at Great Lakes Conference, September 30, 2006; M. F. McCarty, "High Dose Pyridoxine as an Anti-stress Strategy," *Medical Hypotheses* 54 (2000): 803–807.

11. D. Mischoulon and M. F. Raab, "The Role of Folate in Depression and Dementia: Review Article," *Journal of Clinical Psychiatry*, Supplement 68, no. 10 (2007): 28–33.

12. J. J. Cannell, "Autism and Vitamin D," *Medical Hypotheses* 70, no. 4 (2008): 750–759.

13. W. A. Hoogendijk et al., "Depression Is Associated with Decreased 25-Hydroxyvitamin D and Increased Parathyroid Hormone Levels in Older Adults," *Archives of General Psychiatry* 65, no. 5 (2008): 508–512; A. Huotari and K. H. Herzig, "Vitamin D and Living in Northern Latitudes—An Endemic Risk Area for Vitamin D Deficiency," *International Journal of Circumpolar Health* 67 (June 2008): 164–178.

14. E. Garcion et al., "New Clues About Vitamin D Functions in the Nervous System," *Trends in Endocrinology and Metabolism* 13, no. 3 (2002): 100–105.

15. Y. Zhang et al., "AKT Pathway Is Activated by 1, 25-Hydroxyvitamin D_3 and Participates in Its Anti-Apoptotic Effect and Cell Cycle Control in HL60 Cells," *Cell Cycle* 5, no. 4 (2006): 447–451.

16. N. Binkley et al., "Low Vitamin D Status Despite Abundant Sun Exposure," *Journal of Clinical Endocrinology and Metabolism* 92, no. 6 (2007): 2130–2135.

17. D. Mischoulon, "Update and Critique of Natural Remedies as Antidepressant Treatments," *Psychiatric Clinics of North America* 30 (2007): 51–68.

18. J. Lombard, "Neurobiology of Mood and Cognition: Strategies and Protocols of Neurotransmitter Balance," presented at Great Lakes Conference, September 30, 2006.

19. M. Maes et al., "Lower Serum Zinc in Major Depression in Relation to Changes in Serum Acute Phase Proteins," *Journal of Affective Disorders* 56, no. 2 (1999): 189–194.

20. S. Barrondo et al., "Allosteric Modulation of 5-HT(1A) Receptors by Zinc: Binding Studies," *Neuropharmacology* 56, no. 2 (2009): 455–462; A. S. Nakashima and R. H. Dyck, "Zinc and Cortical Plasticity," *Brain Research Reviews* 59 (2009): 347–373.

21. V. Darbinyan et al., "Clinical Trial of *Rhodiola rosea* L. Extract SHR-5 in the Treatment of Mild to Moderate Depression," *Nordic Journal of Psychiatry* 61, no. 5 (2007): 343–348.

22. A. Bystritsky et al., "A Pilot Study of *Rhodiola rosea* (Rhodax) for Generalized Anxiety Disorder (GAD)," *Journal of Alternative and Complementary Medicine* 14, no. 2 (2008): 175–180.

23. F. Khanum et al., "*Rhodiola rosea*: A Versatile Adaptogen," *Comprehensive Reviews in Food Science and Food Safety* 4 (2005): 55–62.

24. J. Lombard, "Neurobiology of Mood and Cognition: Strategies and Protocols of Neurotransmitter Balance," presented at Great Lakes Conference, September 30, 2006.

25. K. Kobayashi et al., "Effects of L-Theanine on the Release of Alpha-Brain Waves in Human Volunteers," *Journal of the Agricultural Chemical Society of Japan* 72, no. 2 (1998): 153–157.

26. J. Lake, "Integrative Management of Anxiety," *Psychiatric Times* 25, no. 1 (January 2008): 13–16.

27. J. Grant et al., "N-Acetyl Cysteine, a Glutamate-Modulating Agent, in the Treatment of Pathological Gambling: A Pilot Study," *Biological Psychiatry* 62, no. 6 (2007): 652–657; J. Grant et al., "N-Acetylcysteine, a Glutamate Modulator, in the Treatment of Trichotillomania," *Archives of General Psychiatry* 66, no. 7 (July 2009): 756–763.

28. www.med.yale.edu/psych/clinics/OCD%20Research%20Clinic/N-acetycysteine .htm.

29. M. Mori et al., "Beta-Alanine and Taurine as Endogenous Agonists at Glycine Receptors in Rat Hippocampus *in Vitro*," *Journal of Physiology* 539 (2002): 191–200; H. Wu et al., "Mode of Action of Taurine as a Neuroprotector," *Brain Research* 1038, no. 2 (March 2005): 123–131.

30. A. Palatnik et al., "Double Blind, Controlled, Crossover Trial of Inositol Versus Fluvoxamine for the Treatment of Panic Disorder," *Journal of Clinical Psychopharmacology* 21, no. 3 (2001): 335–339.

31. A. Abdou et al., "Relaxation and Immunity Enhancement Effects of Gamma-Aminobutyric Acid (GABA) Administration in Humans," *BioFactors* 26 (2006): 201–208.

32. M. Robichaud and G. Debonnel, "Modulation of the Firing Activity of Female Dorsal Raphe Nucleus Serotonergic Neurons by Neuroactive Steroids," *Journal of Endocrinology* 182 (2004): 11–21; R. Genud et al., "DHEA Lessens Depressive-Like Behavior via GABA-ergic Modulation of the Mesolimbic System," *Neuropsychopharmacology* 34 (2009): 577–584.

33. G. Kinrys et al., "Natural Remedies for Anxiety Disorders: Potential Use and Clinical Applications," *Depression and Anxiety* 26 (2009): 259–265.

34. S. Akhondzadeh et al., "Passionflower in the Treatment of Generalized Anxiety Disorder: A Pilot Double-Blind Randomized Controlled Trial with Oxazepam," *Journal of Clinical Pharmacy and Therapeutics* 26 (2001): 363–367.

35. C. S. Yuan et al., "The Gamma-aminobutyric Acidergic Effects of Valerian and Valerenic Acid on Rat Brainstem Neuronal Activity," *Anesthesia and Analgesia* 98 (2004): 353–358.

36. M. Panijel, "Therapy of Symptoms of Anxiety," *Therapiewoche* 41 (1985): 4659–4668.

37. R. Teufel-Mayer and J. Sleitz, "Effects of Long-Term Administration of Hypericum Extracts on the Affinity and Density of the Central Serotonergic 5-HT1 A and 5-HT2 A Receptors," *Pharmacopsychiatry* 30 (1997): 113–116; B. Thiele et al., "Modulation of Cytokine Expression by Hypericum Extract," *Nevenheilkunde* 12 (1993): 353–356.

38. T. Davidson and K. M. Connor, "St. John's Wort in Generalized Anxiety Disorder: Three Case Reports," *Journal of Clinical Psychopharmacology* 21 (2001): 635–636; L. Taylor and K. Kobak, "An Open-Label Trial of St. John's Wort (*Hypericum perforatum*) in Obsessive-Compulsive Disorder," *Journal of Clinical Psychiatry* 61 (2000): 575–578.

39. A. Walesiuk et al., "*Ginkgo biloba* Normalizes Stress- and Corticosterone-induced Impairment of Recall in Rats," *Pharmacological Research* 53 (2006): 123–128.

40. H. Woelk et al., "*Ginkgo biloba* Special Extract EGb761 in Generalized Anxiety Disorder and Adjustment Disorder with Anxious Mood: A Randomized, Double-Blind, Placebo Controlled Trial," *Journal of Psychiatric Research* 41 (2007): 472–480.

Chapter 6: Manage Your Energy

1. R. A. Rizza et al., "Cortisol-Induced Insulin Resistance in Man: Impaired Suppression of Glucose Production and Stimulation of Glucose Utilization Due to a Postreceptor Defect of Insulin Action," *Journal of Clinical Endocrinology and Metabolism* 54 (1982): 131–138.

2. M. E. Gluck et al., "Cortisol Stress Response Is Positively Correlated with Central Obesity in Obese Women with Binge Eating Disorder (BED) Before and After Cognitive-Behavioral Treatment," *Annals of the New York Academy of Sciences* 1032 (2004): 202–207.

3. R. S. Ahima and J. S. Flier, "Adipose Tissue as an Endocrine Organ," *Trends in Endocrinology and Metabolism* 11, no. 8 (2000): 327–332.

4. R. C. Andrews and B. R. Walker, "Glucocorticoids and Insulin Resistance: Old Hormones, New Targets," *Clinical Science* 96 (1999): 513–523.

5. www.nhlbi.nih.gov/health/dci/Diseases/ms/ms_whatis.html.

6. H. Koponen et al., "Metabolic Syndrome Predisposes to Depressive Symptoms: A Population-Based 7-Year Follow-Up Study," *Journal of Clinical Psychiatry* 69, no. 2 (2008): 178–182.

7. M. R. Irwin and A. H. Miller, "Depressive Disorders and Immunity: 20 Years of Progress and Discovery," *Brain, Behavior and Immunity* 21, no. 4 (2007): 374–383.

8. A. Reichenberg et al., "Cytokine-Associated Emotional and Cognitive Disturbances in Humans," *Archives of General Psychiatry* 58, no. 5 (May 2001): 445–452; R. S. Duman and L. M. Monteggia, "A Neurotrophic Model for Stress-Related Mood Disorders," *Biological Psychiatry* 59, no. 12 (2006): 1116–1127.

9. J. H. O'Keefe et al., "Dietary Strategies for Improving Post-Prandial Glucose, Lipids, Inflammation, and Cardiovascular Health," *Journal of the American College of Cardiology* 51 (2008): 249–255.

10. B. Qin et al., "Cinnamon Extract (Traditional Herb) Potentiates *in Vivo* Insulin-Regulated Glucose Utilization Via Enhancing Insulin Signaling in Rats," *Diabetes Research and Clinical Practice* 62, no. 3 (2003): 139–148.

11. E. Ostman et al., "Vinegar Supplementation Lowers Glucose and Insulin Responses and Increases Satiety After a Bread Meal in Healthy Subjects," *European Journal of Clinical Nutrition* 59 (2005): 983–988.

12. B. H. Ali et al., "Some Phytochemical, Pharmacological and Toxicological Properties of Ginger (*Zingiber officinale* Roscoe): A Review of Recent Research," *Food and Chemical Toxicology* 46, no. 2 (2008): 409–420; N. Chainani-Wu, "Safety and Anti-Inflammatory Activity of Curcumin: A Component of Turmeric (*Curcuma longa*)," *Journal of Alternative and Complementary Medicine* 9, no. 1 (2003): 161–168.

13. A. Midaoui and J. de Champlain, "Prevention of Hypertension, Insulin Resistance and Oxidative Stress by Alpha-Lipoic Acid," *Hypertension* 39 (2002): 303–307.

14. J. Liu et al., "Age-Associated Mitochondrial Oxidative Decay: Improvement of Carnitine Acetyltransferase Substrate-Binding Affinity and Activity in Brain by Feeding Old Rats Acetyl-l-Carnitine and/or R-alpha-Lipoic Acid," *Proceedings of the National Academy of Sciences of the United States of America* 99, no. 4 (2002): 1876–1881.

15. R. T. Mathews et al., "Coenzyme Q_{10} Administration Increases Brain Mitochondrial Concentrations and Exerts Neuroprotective Effects," *Proceedings of the National Academy of Sciences of the United States of America* 95, no. 15 (1998): 8892–8897.

16. J. G. Seifert et al., "The Role of Ribose on Oxidative Stress During Hypoxic Exercise: A Pilot Study," *Journal of Medicinal Food* 12, no. 3 (2009): 690–693.

17. L. Wu et al., "Green Tea Supplementation Ameliorates Insulin Resistance and Increases Glucose Transporter IV Content in a Fructose-Fed Rat Model," *European Journal of Nutrition* 43, no. 2 (2004): 116–124; G. W. Varilek et al., "Green Tea Polyphenol Extract Attenuates Inflammation in Interleukin-2-Deficient Mice, a Model of Autoimmunity," *Journal of Nutrition* 131 (2001): 2034–2039.

18. J. Shi et al., "Polyphenolics in Grape Seeds—Biochemistry and Functionality," *Journal of Medicinal Food* 6, no. 4 (2004): 291–299.

19. L. Packer et al., "Antioxidant Activity and Biologic Properties of a Procyanidin-Rich Extract from Pine (*Pinus maritime*) Bark, Pycnogenol," *Free Radical Biology and Medicine* 27 (1999): 704–724.

20. V. Vuksan et al., "Beneficial Effects of Viscous Dietary Fiber from Konjac-mannan in Subjects with Insulin Resistance Syndrome: Results of a Controlled Metabolic Trial," *Diabetes Care* 23, no. 1 (2000): 9–14.

21. J. P. Docherty et al., "A Double-Blind, Placebo-Controlled, Exploratory Trial of Chromium Picolinate in Atypical Depression: Effect on Carbohydrate Craving," *Journal of Psychiatric Practice* 11, no. 5 (2005): 302–314.

22. J. C. Lovejoy, "The Influence of Dietary Fat on Insulin Resistance," *Current Diabetes Reports* 2, no. 5 (2002): 435–440.

23. Y. Xu et al., "Curcumin Reverses Impaired Hippocampal Neurogenesis and Increases Serotonin Receptor 1A mRNA and Brain-Derived Neurotrophic Factor Expression in Chronically Stressed Rats," *Brain Research* 1162 (2007): 9–18; A. Wu et al., "Dietary Curcumin Counteracts the Outcome of Traumatic Brain Injury on Oxidative Stress, Synaptic Plasticity and Cognition," *Experimental Neurology* 197, no. 2 (2006): 309–317.

24. J. B. Bartholomew et al., "Effects of Acute Exercise on Mood and Well-Being in Patients with Major Depressive Disorder," *Medicine and Science in Sports and Exercise* 37, no. 12 (2005): 2032–2037.

25. J. A. Blumenthal et al., "Exercise and Pharmacotherapy in the Treatment of Major Depressive Disorder," *Psychosomatic Medicine* 69 (2007): 587–596; M. H.

Trivedi et al., "Exercise as an Augmentation Strategy for Treatment of Major Depression," *Journal of Psychiatric Practice* 12, no. 4 (2006): 205–213.

26. J. J. Broman-Fulks et al., "Effects of Aerobic Exercise on Anxiety Sensitivity," *Behaviour Research and Therapy* 42, no. 2 (2004): 125–136.

27. S. A. Anderssen et al., "Combined Diet and Exercise Intervention Reverses the Metabolic Syndrome in Middle-Aged Males: Results from the Oslo Diet and Exercise Study," *Scandinavian Journal of Medicine and Science in Sports*, 17, no. 6 (2007): 687–695.

28. L. Byberg et al., "Total Mortality After Changes in Leisure Time Physical Activity in 50 Year Old Men: 35 Year Follow-Up of Population Based Cohort," *British Medical Journal* 338 (2009): b668.

29. J. G. Hunsberger et al., "Antidepressant Actions of the Exercise-Regulated Gene VGF," *Nature Medicine* 13 (2007): 1476–1482.

30. J. S. Snyder et al., "The Effects of Exercise and Stress on the Survival and Maturation of Adult-Generated Granule Cells," *Hippocampus*, epub ahead of print (January 20, 2009): 1–9; B. Winter et al., "High-Impact Running Improves Learning," *Neurobiology of Learning and Memory* 87, no. 4 (2007): 597–609.

31. S. Vaynman and F. Gomez-Pinilla, "License to Run: Exercise Impacts Functional Plasticity in the Intact and Injured Central Nervous System by Using Neurotrophins," *Neurorehabilitation and Neural Repair* 19, no. 4 (2005): 283–295.

32. B. Liebman, "Chair Today, Gone Tomorrow," interview with James Levine, MD, *Nutrition Action Healthletter* 35, no. 3 (April 2008): 3–6.

Chapter 7: Align with Nature

1. P. A. Levine, *Waking the Tiger: Healing Trauma: The Innate Capacity to Transform Overwhelming Experiences* (Berkeley: North Atlantic Books, 1997).

2. G. Paul et al., "A Longitudinal Study of Students' Perceptions of Using Deep Breathing Meditation to Reduce Testing Stress," *Teaching and Learning in Medicine* 19, no. 3 (2007): 287–292.

3. A. Conrad et al., "Psychophysiological Effects of Breathing Instructions for Stress Management," *Applied Psychophysiology and Biofeedback* 32 (2007): 89–98.

4. M. Kundera, as quoted in D. Gelbert, *The Canine Hiker's Bible* (Montchanen, DE: Cruden Bay Books, 2004).

5. www.quotationspage.com/quote/1735.html.

6. A. N. Vgontzas et al., "Chronic Insomnia Is Associated with Nyctohemeral Activation of the Hypothalamic-Pituitary-Adrenal Axis: Clinical Implications," *Journal of Clinical Endocrinology and Metabolism* 86, no. 8 (2001): 3787–3794.

7. National Institutes of Health, National Center on Sleep Disorders Research, *2003 National Sleep Disorders Research Plan*, U.S. Department of Health and Human Services, 2003.

Chapter 8: Quiet the Mind

1. P. Chodron, *Bodhisattva Mind: Teachings to Cultivate Courage and Awareness in the Midst of Suffering* (Boulder: Sounds True, 2006).
2. Ibid.

Chapter 9: Turn Toward the Feeling

1. S. Young, *Break Through Difficult Emotions: How to Transform Painful Feelings with Mindfulness Meditation* (Boulder: Sounds True, 1997).
2. P. Chodron, *Boddhisattva Mind: Teachings to Cultivate Courage and Awareness in the Midst of Suffering* (Boulder: Sounds True, 2006).

Chapter 10: Cultivate a Good Heart

1. T. Brach, *Radical Acceptance: Embracing Your Life With the Heart of a Buddha* (New York: Bantam Books, 2004).
2. R. Davidson, "Anxiety and Affective Style: Role of Prefrontal Cortex and Amygdala," *Biological Psychiatry* 51 (2002): 68–80.
3. www.medicine.indiana.edu/news_releases/archive_02/violent_games02.html.
4. A. Lutz et al., "Regulation of the Neural Circuitry of Emotion by Compassion Meditation: Effects of Meditative Expertise," *PLoS One* 3, no. 3 (2008): e1897.

Chapter 11: Create Deep Connections

1. *The Tao Te Ching*, trans. S. Mitchell (New York: Harper, 1992).
2. L. Cozolino, *The Neuroscience of Human Relations* (New York: Norton, 2006).
3. www.examiner.com/x-6495-US-Intelligence-Examiner~y2009m8d24 -Educational-documentary-Japanese-school-teacher-transforms-students.
4. M. Oliver, *New and Selected Poems*, vol. 1 (Boston: Beacon Press, 1992).
5. J. Tarrant, *The Light Inside the Dark: Zen, Soul and the Spiritual Life* (New York: Harper, 1999).

Chapter 12: The Science of Hope

1. W. James, *Principles of Psychology*, vol. 1 (London: Macmillan, 1890): 108.
2. E. Lugaro, "Le Resistenze nell'evoluzione della vita," *Rivista Moderna di Cultura* 1 (1898): 29–60.
3. D. O. Hebb, *The Organization of Behavior: A Neuropsychological Theory* (New York: Wiley, 1949): 70.
4. S. F. Cooke and T. V. Bliss, "Plasticity in the Human Central Nervous System," *Brain* 129 (2006): 1659–1673.
5. A. Pascual-Leone et al., "Modulation of Muscle Responses Evoked by

Transcranial Magnetic Stimulation During the Acquisition of New Fine Motor Skills," *Journal of Neurophysiology* 74 (1995): 1037–1045.

6. J. M. Schwartz et al., "Systematic Changes in Cerebral Glucose Metabolic Rate After Successful Behavior Modification Treatment of Obsessive-Compulsive Disorder," *Archives of General Psychiatry* 53 (1996): 109–113.

7. J. M. Schwartz, "Neuroanatomical Aspects of Cognitive-Behavioural Therapy Response in Obsessive-Compulsive Disorder: An Evolving Perspective on Brain and Behaviour," *British Journal of Psychiatry,* Supplement 35 (1998): 38–44.

8. K. Felmingham, A. Kemp, et al., "Changes in Anterior Cingulate and Amygdala After Cognitive Behavior Therapy of Post-Traumatic Stress Disorder," *Psychological Science* 18, no. 2 (2007): 127–129.

9. V. Paquette et al., " 'Change the Mind and You Change the Brain': Effects of Cognitive Behavioral Therapy on the Neural Correlates of Spider Phobia," *NeuroImage* 18 (2003): 401–409.

10. R. J. Davidson, "Emotion and Affective Style: Hemispheric Substrates," *Psychological Science* 3 (1992): 39–43.

11. R. J. Davidson et al., "Alterations in Brain and Immune Function Produced by Mindfulness Meditation," *Psychosomatic Medicine* 65 (2003): 564–570.

12. A. Lutz et al., "Long-term Meditators Self-Induce High Amplitude Gamma Synchrony During Mental Practice," *Proceedings of the National Academy of Sciences* 101, no. 46 (November 16, 2004): 16369–16373.

13. S. A. Goldman and F. Nottebohm, "Neuronal Production, Migration and Differentiation in Control Nucleus of the Adult Female Canary Brain," *Proceedings of the National Academy of Sciences USA* 80 (April 1983): 2390–2394.

14. P. S. Eriksson et al., "Neurogenesis in the Adult Human Hippocampus," *Nature Medicine* 4, no. 11 (November 1998): 1313–1317.

15. E. J. Huang and L. F. Reichart, "Neurotrophins: Roles in Neuronal Development and Function," *Annual Review of Neuroscience* 24 (March 2001): 677–736.

16. X. Jiang et al., "BDNF Variation and Mood Disorders: A Novel Functional Promoter Polymorphism and Val66Met Are Associated with Anxiety but Have Opposing Effects," *Neuropsychopharmacology* 30 (2005): 1353–1361; H. S. Phillips et al., "BDNF mRNA Is Decreased in the Hippocampus of Individual with Alzheimer's Disease," *Neuron* 7, no. 5 (November 1991): 695–702; D. W. Howells et al., "Reduced BDNF mRNA Expression in the Parkinson's Disease Substantia Nigra," *Experimental Neurology* 166, no. 1 (November 2000): 127–135.

17. J. L. Warner-Schmidt and R. S. Duman, "Hippocampal Neurogenesis: Opposing Effects of Stress and Antidepressant Treatment," *Hippocampus* 16, no. 3 (2006): 239–249.

18. D. O. Hebb, "The Effects of Early Experience on Problem-Solving at Maturity," *American Psychologist* 2 (1947): 306–307.

19. M. R. Rosenzweig and E. L. Bennett, "Effects of Differential Environments on Brain Weights and Enzyme Activities in Gerbils, Rats, and Mice," *Developmental Psychobiology* 2 (1969): 87–95.

20. G. Kempermann et al., "More Hippocampal Neurons in Adult Mice Living in an Enriched Environment," *Nature* 386 (1997): 493–495.

21. G. Kempermann et al., "Experience-Induced Neurogenesis in the Senescent Dentate Gyrus," *Journal of Neuroscience* 18 (1998): 3206–3212.

22. H. van Praag et al., "Running Increases Cell Proliferation and Neurogenesis in the Adult Mouse Dentate Gyrus," *Nature Neuroscience* 2 (1999): 266–270.

23. A. Garza et al., "Exercise, Antidepressant Treatment, and BDNF mRNA Expression in the Aging Brain," *Pharmacology, Biochemistry and Behavior* 77, no. 2 (2004): 209–220.

24. B. Eadie et al., "Voluntary Exercise Increases Neurogenic Activity in the Dentate Gyrus of the Adult Mammalian Brain: Fact or Fiction?" poster presented at the annual meeting of the Society for Neuroscience, 2004.

25. H. Soya et al., "BDNF Induction with Mild Exercise in the Rat Hippocampus," *Biochemical and Biophysical Research Communications* 358, no. 4 (2007): 961–967.

26. J. Currie et al., "Cardio-Respiratory Fitness, Habitual Physical Activity and Serum Brain Derived Neurotrophic Factor (BDNF) in Men and Women," *Neuroscience Letter* 451, no. 2 (2009): 152–155.

27. S. Rojas Vegas et al., "Acute BDNF and Cortisol Response to Low Intensity Exercise and Following Ramp Incremental Exercise to Exhaustion in Humans," *Brain Research* 1121, no. 1 (2006): 59–65.

28. J. Lee et al., "Dietary Restriction Increases the Number of Newly Generated Neural Cells, and Induces BDNF Expression, in the Dentate Gyrus of Rats," *Journal of Molecular Neuroscience* 15, no. 2 (2000): 99–108.

29. C. M. Williams et al., "Blueberry-Induced Changes in Spatial Working Memory Correlate with Changes in Hippocampal CREB Phosphorylation and Brain-Derived Neurotrophic Factor (BDNF) Levels," *Free Radical Biology and Medicine*, 45, no. 3 (2008): 295–305.

30. K. L. Chan et al., "Relationship of Serum Brain-Derived Neurotrophic Factor (BDNF) and Health-Related Lifestyle in Healthy Human Subjects," *Neuroscience Letter* 447 (2008): 124–128.

31. A. Wu et al., "Dietary Omega-3 Fatty Acids Normalize BDNF Levels, Reduce Oxidative Damage, and Counteract Learning Disability After Traumatic Brain Injury in Rats," *Journal of Neurotrauma* 21, no. 10 (2004): 1457–1467.

32. M. P. Mattson et al., "BDNF and 5-HT: A Dynamic Duo in Age-Related Neuronal Plasticity and Neurodegenerative Disorders," *Trends in Neuroscience* 27, no. 10 (2004): 589–594.

33. A. A. Garza et al., "Exercise, Antidepressant Treatment, and BDNF mRNA Expression in the Aging Brain," *Pharmacology Biochemistry & Behavior* 77 (2004): 209–20.

34. A. Strasser et al., "The Impact of Environment in Comparison with Moderate Physical Exercise and Dietary Restriction on BDNF in the Cerebral Parieto-temporal Cortex of Aged Sprague-Dawley Rats," *Gerontology* 52, no. 6 (2006): 377–381.

35. M. F. Fraga et al., "Epigenetic Differences Arise During the Lifetime of Mono-zygotic Twins," *Proceedings of the National Academy of Science, USA* 102 (2005): 10604–10609.

36. A. Bergmann and M. E. Lane, "Hidden Targets of MicroRNAs for Growth Control," *Trends in Biochemical Science* 28 (2003): 461–463.

37. J. C. Mathers, "Personalized Nutrition Epigenomics: A Basis for Understanding Individual Differences?" *Proceedings of the Nutrition Society* 67 (2008): 390–394.

38. R. A. Waterland and R. L. Jirtle, "Transposable Elements: Targets for Early Nutritional Effects on Epigenetic Gene Regulation," *Molecular Cell Biology* 23 (2003): 5293–5300.

39. K. D. Sinclair et al., "DNA Methylation, Insulin Resistance and Blood Pressure in Offspring Determined by Maternal Periconceptional B Vitamin and Methionine Status," *Proceedings of the National Academy of Science, USA* 104 (2007): 19351–19356.

40. S. Friso et al., "A Common Mutation in the 5, 10-Methylenetetrahydrofolate-Reductase Gene Affects Genomic DNA Methylation Through an Interaction with Folate Status," *Proceedings of the National Academy of Science, USA* 99 (2002): 5605–5611.

41. D. Liu et al., "Maternal Care, Hippocampal Glucocorticoid Receptors, and Hypothalamic-Pituitary-Adrenal Responses to Stress," *Science* 277 (1997): 1659–1662.

42. I. C. G. Weaver et al., "Epigenetic Programming by Maternal Behavior," *Nature and Neuroscience* 7 (2004): 847–854.

43. Ibid.

44. T. Hayashi et al., "Laughter Regulates Gene Expression in Type 2 Diabetes," *Psychotherapy and Psychosomatics* 75, no. 1 (2006): 62–65.

45. J. A. Dusek et al., "Genomic Counter-Stress Changes Induced by the Relaxation Response," *PLoS One* 3, no. 7 (2008): e2576.

46. A. P. Feinberg, "Phenotypic Plasticity and the Epigenetics of Human Disease," *Nature* 447 (2007): 433–440.

Afterword: The Call to Courage

1. S. Lebell, Epictetus, *The Art of Living: The Classic Manual on Virtue, Happiness and Effectiveness* (New York: Harper One, 2004).

2. D. Ladinsky, *The Subject Tonight Is Love: 60 Wild and Sweet Poems of Hafiz* (New York: Penguin Compass, 2003).

Index

abdominal fat, 11, 107, 108–9
acetyl L-carnitine, 114, 116
adrenal glands, 9, 95, 147
adrenaline (epinephrine), 77, 95
alcohol, 28, 29, 145–46, 147
alpha-lipoic acid, 114, 116
amino acids, 65, 66
  arginine, 97
  GABA, *see* GABA
  L-theanine, 75–78, 89–91, 94, 143,
    147, 148
  neurotransmitters and, 74
  taurine, 74, 75, 76, 89, 93
  tryptophan, 66, 75, 79, 91, 143
  in valerian, 97
amygdala, 45, 76, 236
antibiotics, 60, 66
antidepressants, 30
antioxidants, 62, 63, 105, 106, 112, 117,
  244
  acetyl L-carnitine, 114, 116
  alpha-lipoic acid, 114, 116
  grapeseed extract, 115, 117
  green tea, 59, 70, 74, 76, 89, 90, 115,
    117
  glutathione, 92
  NAC, 74–77, 89, 92–93
  pycnogenol, 115, 117
  supplemental, 62, 63, 75, 76, 89,
    92–93, 115, 117

turmeric extract (curcumin), 113,
  116, 117
anxiety, 5–8, 11, 18–31, 55
  bottom-up, 38, 39–41
  evolution and, 21–22
  5-HTP and, 89
  ginkgo and, 98
  hysteria, 25–26
  inflammation and, 10
  inositol and, 93
  L-theanine and, 91
  medications to alleviate, 28–31
  muddled-middle, 38, 44–47
  passionflower and, 96
  St. John's wort and, 97
  seven types of, 38–47
  sleep and, 143
  in soldiers, 22–25
  top-down, 38, 41–44
  valerian and, 97
arginine, 97
Aristotle, 101
arrow metaphor, 12, 153–54
Ativan, 29, 73, 96
ATP, 104, 114, 115
attachment:
  to experience, 185–86
  practicing non-attachment to
    emotion, 190–93
aversion, 185–86, 199

271

About the Author

HENRY EMMONS, M.D., is a psychiatrist who integrates mind-body and natural therapies, mindfulness and allied Buddhist therapeutics, and psychotherapeutic caring and insight in his clinical work. Dr. Emmons obtained his medical degree from the University of Iowa College of Medicine and did his residency in psychiatry at the University of Rochester Medical Center, where he was chief resident. Dr. Emmons is in demand as a workshop and retreat leader for both health care professionals and the general public. He practices general and holistic psychiatry and consults to several colleges and organizations nationally. He currently serves as consulting psychiatrist at the Penny George Institute for Health and Healing in Minneapolis, Minnesota.